ACUTE RESPIRATORY
FAILURE IN THE ADULT

NEW ENGLAND JOURNAL OF MEDICINE
MEDICAL PROGRESS SERIES

ACUTE RESPIRATORY FAILURE IN THE ADULT

HENNING PONTOPPIDAN, M.D.

ASSOCIATE PROFESSOR OF ANAESTHESIA, HARVARD MEDICAL
SCHOOL AT THE MASSACHUSETTS GENERAL HOSPITAL;
CHIEF, RESPIRATORY UNIT, AND ANESTHETIST,
MASSACHUSETTS GENERAL HOSPITAL, BOSTON

BENNIE GEFFIN, M.D.

ASSISTANT PROFESSOR OF ANAESTHESIA, HARVARD MEDICAL
SCHOOL AT THE MASSACHUSETTS GENERAL HOSPITAL;
ASSOCIATE ANESTHETIST, MASSACHUSETTS GENERAL HOSPITAL, BOSTON

EDWARD LOWENSTEIN, M.D.

ASSOCIATE PROFESSOR OF ANAESTHESIA, HARVARD MEDICAL
SCHOOL AT THE MASSACHUSETTS GENERAL HOSPITAL;
CHIEF, CARDIAC ANESTHESIA GROUP, AND ANESTHETIST,
MASSACHUSETTS GENERAL HOSPITAL, BOSTON

LITTLE, BROWN AND COMPANY

BOSTON

This monograph is expanded from ma-
terial which first appeared as a Medical
Progress Report in the *New England
Journal of Medicine.*

Printed in the United States of America

PREFACE

ORGANIZED systems for the management of patients with acute respiratory failure first evolved during the poliomyelitis epidemics of the early and middle 1950s. Their obvious success stimulated considerable interest in acutely ill patients and resulted in the development of the first intensive care units oriented predominantly toward their respiratory problems.

With accumulated experience and improved survival data, it has become apparent that multisystem failure is the rule in critically ill patients. The current trend is, therefore, toward the development of generalized intensive care units where derangements of all systems can be observed and managed. While respiratory failure remains a fundamental common denominator—and the present review is designed to focus primarily on this aspect of critical care medicine—it is necessary also to emphasize the indispensable role of cardiovascular and renal assessment and therapy in patients with acute respiratory failure.

This publication is an expanded and slightly revised version of a three-part Medical Progress Report published in the *New England Journal of Medicine* in late 1972. It is intended for all physicians interested in the care of critically ill patients, and supplements and brings up to date a previous publication (*Respiratory Care*) from our department. Throughout we have emphasized the application of physiologic concepts and data to the clinical setting.

The topics considered deal with those areas in which we believe progress has most notably contributed to a better understanding of, and improved outlook for, patients with acute respiratory failure. The inevitable limitations of space have made it impossible for important topics such as improved antibiotic therapy, intravenous hyperalimentation and membrane oxygenation to be included.

The material presented reflects our experience at the Massachusetts General Hospital. Appropriately, care has been predominantly a team effort. To the patients' primary physicians, we express our gratitude for their confidence and support.

We are grateful to Drs. Leroy D. Vandam and Myron B. Laver for their helpful suggestions and critical review of the manuscript.

The project was supported by grants GM-15904-03 and GM-15904-04 from the National Institute of General Medical Sciences.

H. P.
B. G.
E. L.

CONTENTS

Contents

Contents

NOTATIONS USED

ARF: acute respiratory failure
C (a-vDO₂):   arteriovenous oxygen difference
CPPB: continuous positive-pressure breathing
CVP: central venous pressure
FEV_1:   first-second vital capacity
F_IO_2:   inspired oxygen concentration
FRC: functional residual capacity
IPPV: intermittent positive-pressure ventilation
MEFR: maximum expiratory flow rate
$P(A-aDO_2)$:   alveolar-arterial oxygen gradient
$Paco_2$:   arterial carbon dioxide tension
$PAco_2$:   alveolar carbon dioxide tension
Pao_2:   arterial oxygen tension
P_{AO_2}:   alveolar oxygen tension
PEEP: positive end-expiratory pressure
PEVW: pulmonary extravascular water content
$\dot{Q}_S/\dot{Q}_T$: right-to-left shunt
$\dot{V}_A/\dot{Q}$:   ventilation-perfusion ratio
$\dot{V}co_2$:   carbon dioxide production
V_D/V_T: ratio of dead space to tidal volume
$\dot{V}_E$:   minute ventilation

1

GENERAL CONSIDERATIONS

Trends in Treatment of Acute Respiratory Failure

FOR several years after paralytic poliomyelitis became a rare disease, the use of artificial ventilation in treatment of acute respiratory failure was infrequent. During the past decade this trend has rapidly changed.[1] The yearly number of patients treated with prolonged artificial ventilation at the Massachusetts General Hospital, which in 1958 amounted to 66, is now 1400 to 1500. In 1971 such cases accounted for 7230 patient days. Over the past decade more than 7000 patients have been so treated.

Where and by whom should the burgeoning number of patients requiring artificial ventilation be managed? This question, which is inseparable from the larger question of organization of critical-care medicine, is now widely debated,* and there is concern over the high cost of providing adequate care for these patients.† This high cost is a result of the extreme demands on doctors,

---

* For instance, at a conference on "Goal Problems in Intensive Care" held in May, 1971, sponsored by the National Research Council and American College of Surgeons.

† The daily total cost of caring for a patient in the Massachusetts General Hospital Respiratory Unit and Surgical Intensive Care Unit was recently estimated at approximately $500 (Lawrence E. Martin, personal communication, 1972).

nurses and other personnel by the critically ill patients, who need constant nursing care, cannot be left unattended and require immediate availability and often prolonged, constant attention by physicians experienced in critical-care medicine. Although selected patients can best be cared for in the large medical centers with special facilities, to transfer all such patients is impractical, if for no other reason than the sheer numbers involved. This problem must be solved on a regional basis with appropriate community hospitals being designated, equipped and staffed to provide care of the critically ill patient and acting as the regional referral centers.[2,3] A rational solution would be facilitated by improved data on need for critical care and on the short-term and long-term outlook for these patients.

Definition of ARF

As respiratory complications or disease progress and ventilatory reserve diminishes, respiratory failure eventually sets in. Unfortunately, there is no agreement on how this stage should be defined. Most authors have defined respiratory failure by an arterial oxygen tension (Pao_2) or carbon dioxide tension ($Paco_2$) well outside the normal range—e.g., Pao_2 below 60 or $Paco_2$ above 49 mm of mercury.[4] Since Pao_2 falls with age, and the importance of abnormal arterial blood gases varies much from patient to patient, *we define ARF as a state in which Pao_2 is below the predicted normal range for the patient's age at the prevalent barometric pressure*[5,6] *(in the absence of intracardiac right-to-left shunting), or $Paco_2$ above 50 mm of mercury (not due to respiratory compensation for metabolic alkalemia).* To avoid confusion, it should be said at the onset that the meaning of abnormal blood

2

gases and the therapeutic principles in respiratory failure due to acute exacerbation of severe chronic obstructive pulmonary disease and chronic hypoxemia are not identical to those that apply in patients with ARF with little or no pre-existing lung disease. With considerable oversimplification the current emphasis in treating patients with chronic obstructive pulmonary disease is to delay artificial ventilation as long as possible, taking specific advantage of "controlled oxygen therapy." However, one should not lose sight of the fact that chronic pulmonary disease, even though not severe, predisposes strongly to acute pulmonary complications following surgery and trauma.[7]

Contents of Review

This review is chiefly concerned with management of patients with ARF—that is, patients in whom chronic hypoxemia and hypercapnia are not cardinal features. Such patients form the bulk of those treated with artificial ventilation at the Massachusetts General Hospital[1,7] and its Respiratory Unit.[8] Others have reported a similar patient distribution. For example, in 1970 the multidisciplinary intensive-care unit at Presbyterian University Hospital, Pittsburgh, admitted 977 patients.[9] Only 90 cases were classified as "chronic pulmonary disease." It is noteworthy that despite this, more than 50 per cent of the total admissions required prolonged artificial ventilation.[9] Most of these patients suffered from multiple-organ failure.

The pathophysiology and principles of management of ARF have been described in recent publications.[10,11] Our own experience in these areas was presented in detail in 1965[7] and 1970.[1] The mortality rate of patients

TABLE 1. *Patients in the Respiratory Unit at the Massachusetts General Hospital, October, 1961, to December, 1970.**

DIAGNOSIS	NO. OF PATIENTS	NO. OF SURVIVORS
Open-heart surgery	87	44
Thymectomy	47	47
Other thoracic surgery	105	80
Crushed chest	64	57
Abdominal surgery & nonthoracic trauma	179	78
Neurosurgery & head trauma	69	42
Drug poisoning	73	62
Neuromuscular disease	71	56
Emphysema	43	23
Cardiac failure	12	10
Idiopathic respiratory failure†	49	41
Pneumonia	29	25
Miscellaneous	95	76
Totals	923	641

* Over the years there has been a steady improvement in the survival rate, the mortality in 1970 having fallen to 11 per cent. Most patients required tracheal intubation or tracheostomy & artificial ventilation for a large part of their stay in the Respiratory Unit. The average duration of stay was 18 days. Note that only 5 per cent of the patients had ARF based on chronic obstructive pulmonary disease. However, some degree of chronic obstructive disease was present in several other patients, notably in the open-heart thoracic and abdominal surgical groups. A great preponderance of ARF of nonobstructive origin is characteristic for the total hospital population of patients with respiratory failure.

† Patients in ARF with diffuse infiltrative pulmonary changes of undetermined etiology.

admitted to the Respiratory Unit of the Massachusetts General Hospital during the first years of operation (1961–1965) was 35 to 40 per cent. This figure has fallen steadily even though the admission policy has remained the same and there has been no major change in the class of patients admitted. Currently, the mortality is between 10 and 20 per cent, varying substantially with the type of illness (Table 1). A similar improvement in prognosis of patients with acute respiratory failure has been obtained by others.[12] The fall in mortality rate can be attributed to progress in almost all aspects of respiratory care. However, several areas in which improved physiologic understanding has led to rational therapeutic consequences stand out. These areas, which chapters of this book discuss, are:

Patterns of gas distribution in normal lungs and in ARF.
Interstitial pulmonary edema.
Assessment of respiratory function.
Pulmonary oxygen toxicity.
Current use of artificial ventilation.
Effect of mechanical ventilation on circulation and blood gas exchange.
Complications of tracheal intubation and tracheotomy.

Advances have also been recorded in respiratory care of the infant and child, in whom special physiologic and clinical considerations pertain.[13–17] These will not be reviewed in this book.

Nonspecificity of Response to Injury

Although nondescript syndromes such as "wet" lung, "post-perfusion" lung, "shock" lung and "oxygen-toxicity" lung may be separate clinical entities, their pathologic pictures are nonspecific. Until more is learned about the nature of the changes in pulmonary structure and function, one must treat empirically the two conditions invariably present in ARF: the abnormal pattern

5

of gas distribution, with closure of alveoli or airways, or both; and, secondly, an increase in pulmonary extravascular water, with interstitial edema caused either by pulmonary vascular congestion or by loss of integrity of capillary endothelium, with exudation of plasma into the interstitium. Both conditions tend to become manifest on a regional basis dictated by the effect of gravity on the distribution of ventilation, blood flow and extravascular water.[18,19] They result in a reduction in functional residual capacity, a decrease in pulmonary compliance and mismatching of ventilation and blood flow. These are the hallmarks of ARF.

2

PATTERNS OF GAS DISTRIBUTION AND AIRSPACE CLOSURE

Gas Distribution

RECENT studies using radioactive isotopes, single-breath analysis of expired inert gas concentration and rapid in situ freezing of dog lungs have been instrumental in clarifying regional patterns of ventilation in both normal and pathologic conditions. The influence of gravity on regional lung volume (and alveolar size) and the secondary effects on distribution of inspired gas and tendency to airway closure have been clearly demonstrated.

In upright and lateral positions, the pleural pressure shows a vertical gradient of about 0.3 cm of water per centimeter.[20] This gradient is consistent with the concept that tensions are transmitted through the lung as in a liquid with a specific gravity of 0.3. The pleural pressure gradient, however, is independent of the lung volume (which influences the specific gravity of the lung) and is reduced in half in the head-down position. For these reasons factors other than gravity must have a role in determining the pleural pressure gradient. The most important of these factors presumably is the configuration of the lung.[20]

Since alveolar pressure is the same throughout the

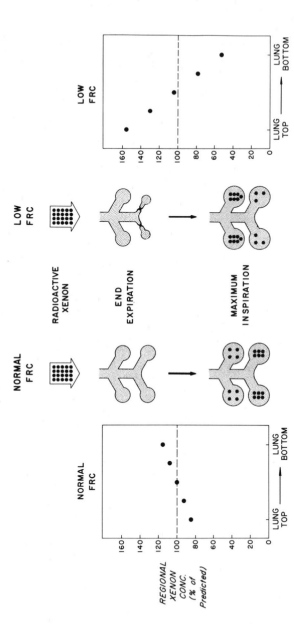

FIGURE 1. *Effect of End-expiratory Regional Lung Volume on Distribution of Inspired Gas* (Reproduced from Pontoppidan et Al. [Edited by Welch][1] with the Permission of Year Book Medical Publishers; Redrawn with Permission from Data of Milici-Emili et Al.[22]).

A bolus of radioactive xenon was inhaled at the beginning of inspiration, and regional radioactivity was measured with counters placed external to the chest at different lung levels. With normal functional residual capacity (FRC), inspired gas is distributed preferentially to the dependent lung region (lung bottom). With a reduction of the FRC and collapse of basal small airways (and possibly also alveoli), the pattern of distribution is reversed, and the nondependent regions will receive a principal portion of the inspired tidal air. Since the dependent lung regions are more highly perfused than the apex, a marked mismatch will occur between ventilation and perfusion. Blood flowing past nonventilated alveoli during the expiratory pause will not be oxygenated properly, and this will contribute to the development of arterial hypoxemia.

lung, gradients in pleural pressure cause regional differences in distending (transpulmonary) pressures. As a consequence of lesser distending pressure, alveoli in dependent lung regions are considerably smaller than superior alveoli. In upright dogs, for instance, this size (volume) differential was fourfold, but the difference in size was reduced as the lung expanded.[21] When lung volume rises, as during inspiration, dependent smaller alveoli represented on the midportion of the S-shaped pressure-volume curve expand more per unit pressure change than superior, large alveoli represented on the upper flat portion of the curve. Thus, during normal breathing, the inspired gas is preferentially distributed to alveoli in the dependent regions, provided the alveoli and airways in this region are open at the beginning of inspiration (Fig. 1).[22] If, on the other hand, dependent alveoli and airways are closed at the beginning of inspiration, inspired gas is preferentially distributed to superior regions since alveoli here increase in size before the critical opening pressure of basal airways is exceeded.[23] Under these circumstances, a reversal of the normal regional ventilation pattern occurs.

Airway Closure and Closing Volume

In the normal person, regardless of age, all regions of the lung are open at the end of a full inspiration. As lung volume decreases during expiration, small airways (0.5 to 0.9 mm in diameter) show a progressive tendency to close,* whereas larger airways remain patent.[25,26] The lung volume at which appreciable small airway closure

---

* It remains to be settled whether closure refers to anatomic airway closure (collapse) or physiologic closure due to dynamic compression,[24] a fluid meniscus, etc.

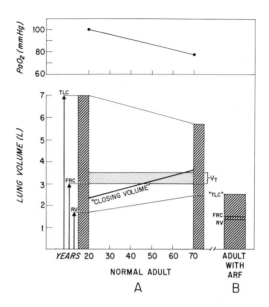

FIGURE 2. *Changes in Pao2 and Lung Volumes with Age in Normal Adults in the Supine Position (A) and Typical Values for FRC and Vital Capacity (B) in an Adult Patient with ARF (RV Represents Residual Volume, FRC Functional Residual Capacity, and TLC Total Lung Capacity).*

The shaded horizontal band represents normal tidal breathing range (V_T). Vital capacity (TLC-RV) falls progressively with age. Closing volume increases linearly with age and in the supine position exceeds FRC at age 44 years. The Pao2 line was drawn from data obtained in supine subjects by Sorbini et al.[6] TLC, RV and FRC are taken from the table of predicted normal values for a male, 175 cm tall, of Bates et al.[11] FRC has been reduced 20 per cent below predicted to account for the fall occurring with change from sitting to supine position. The line indicating closing volume was drawn from data by Leblanc et al.[29]

FRC (B) is greatly reduced, to approximately 50 per cent of predicted. The expiratory reserve column (FRC-RV) is virtually eliminated. Vital capacity, therefore, is primarily inspiratory and is here shown at 1.1 liters—barely consistent with adequate, sustained, spontaneous ventilation.[7] Values are typical for a patient with severe pneumonitis or pulmonary edema. For detailed discussion, see text.

begins is referred to as the closing volume. This volume can be measured by radioactive or inert tracer-gas methods and related to the vital capacity, total lung capacity and the functional residual capacity (FRC) (Fig. 2). Airway closure occurs first in the dependent lung regions, where the distending transpulmonary pressure is less and the volume change during expiration greater.

With advancing age there is an increased tendency toward airspace closure[27] and a progressive linear increase in the closing volume[28,29] (Fig. 2), presumably owing to a progressive decrease in elastic lung recoil. The FRC, on the other hand, remains essentially unchanged with age. As a result, in the upright subject, closing volume exceeds the FRC at 65 years of age. Upon change from upright to supine position, the FRC decreases approximately 20 per cent, whereas the closing volume remains about the same and now exceeds the FRC at a much younger age—namely, 44 years.[29] Airway closure causes gas trapping in alveoli distal to the point of closure. This volume of trapped gas shows a positive correlation with the difference between closing volume and FRC.[30]

During experimental observation in normal subjects, closed units reopen during slow inspiration at a volume only slightly larger than that at which they close during expiration[27]; for practical purposes opening and closing volumes can thus be considered equal. (Opening *pressure*, however, exceeds closing *pressure* due to hysteresis.)

Effect of Airway Closure and Gas Trapping on Gas Exchange

Airway closure affects the regional pattern of gas distribution and results in ventilation-perfusion inequality and impaired blood gas exchange. This presumably accounts for the well-known fact that Pao_2 falls steadily with age (Fig. 2), the greatest fall being in the supine position.[5,6] For the purposes of assessing the effect of airway closure on gas exchange, Craig et al.[31] placed normal subjects, of diverse body build and age, into four groups according to relation of closing volume to FRC and FRC plus tidal volume. Regardless of posture and body build, the greatest impairment in Pao_2, expressed by the alveolar-arterial oxygen tension gradient ($P[\text{A-a}Do_2]$), was observed in subjects whose closing volume exceeded FRC plus tidal volume. Under these circumstances, appreciable airway closure presumably persists throughout inspiration. The $P(\text{A-a}Do_2)$ was minimal in subjects having a closing volume below FRC (Fig. 2). Thus, these investigators concluded that the greater the closing volume in relation to inspiratory lung volume, the more pronounced the effect on gas exchange.

If airways remain closed throughout inspiration, gas trapped in airspaces distal to the point of closure is absorbed by the blood more or less rapidly, according to gas composition and solubility. The end result is atelectasis unless airways are periodically opened by an active or passive deep inspiration. If perfusion continues, venous admixture (shunting) will also occur. Re-expansion of gas-exchanging airspaces may be delayed or refractory because high distending pressures are needed to expand collapsed alveoli. Atelectasis and an increase in $P(\text{A-a}Do_2)$ have, in fact, been reported in normal subjects after breathing at low lung volumes,[32] and a fall in pulmonary compliance evidencing atelectasis was seen after only two minutes of oxygen breathing at low lung volumes (after preceding denitrogenation).[25]

Abnormal Tendency to Airway Closure

In addition to deliberate breathing at low lung volumes, a reduction in FRC and airway closure may come about as a result of other nonpulmonary factors such as the supine[30] and head-down positions and with anesthesia.[33] With obesity[34,35] increased abdominal girth and chest-wall weight reduce lung volume, interfere with proper pulmonary expansion and induce airway closure in dependent lung regions. Any mismatch between blood and gas distribution is then intensified. Abdominal distention, vigorous expiratory effort and suction in the airway may reduce overall lung volume. With inadequate turning of the patient, the same lung regions remain dependent and, therefore, at low lung volumes for prolonged periods. Paralysis, debility, narcotic drugs and pain interfere with spontaneous sighing,[7] which may normally minimize the effect of airway and alveolar closure by intermittently providing the transpulmonary pressure required to open all regions of the lung. Many of these factors are present after surgery, and a reduction in FRC has, in fact, been shown in the postoperative period.[7] Pulmonary factors promoting alveolar and airway closure include increased surface tension, interstitial edema,[36] inflammation with swelling of bronchial or interbronchial tissue and constriction of smooth muscle.

Airway Versus Alveolar Closure

Although the experimental evidence discussed above seems to justify the conclusion that closure of small airways and gas trapping are the predominant sequelae of breathing at low lung volumes, there is evidence that

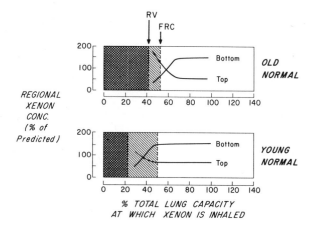

FIGURE 3. *Effect of Age upon Closing Volume* (Reproduced from Pontoppidan et Al. [Edited by Welch][1] with the Permission of the Publisher; Redrawn with Permission from Data of Holland et Al.[27]).

A bolus of radioactive xenon was inhaled during a maximum inspiration, starting from FRC. Regional lung xenon concentrations were monitored during the subsequent expiration with counters placed over the chest. In the elderly, loss of xenon activity is recorded at the base when a volume equivalent to 54 per cent of vital capacity is reached, suggesting alveolar collapse before end-expiration. The apical xenon concentration rises due to a shift of radioactive gas from the base to the apex (crossover of two solid lines). A similar pattern is seen in the young only when expiration is continued below the FRC point. Airway closure in the old individual can be prevented, at least theoretically, by moving the range of tidal ventilation above the crossover point of the Bottom and Top curves, i.e., from approximately 54 to above 60 per cent of total lung capacity (see Fig. 2).

closure of terminal gas-exchanging airspaces also occurs. For example, studies by Holland et al.[27] (Fig. 3), showing a decrease in radioactive xenon concentration over dependent lung regions in the course of an expiratory maneuver, are more consistent with expulsion of gas due to alveolar closure. Airway collapse and gas trapping have also been ruled out as a cause for compliance fall in rabbits and lambs ventilated at shallow tidal volumes.[37]

Lung Volume, Airspace Closure and Oxygenation in ARF

In ARF lung volumes are invariably reduced.[38-40] As FRC falls, expiratory reserve volume is reduced toward zero, and in more severe respiratory failure, the FRC becomes less than predicted residual volume (Fig. 2). Efficiency of oxygenation is closely related to the change in lung volume: in surgical patients FRC and right-to-left shunt ($\dot{Q}_S/\dot{Q}_T$) show a negative correlation,[41] and in a group of patients with respiratory failure, some breathing spontaneously, and others mechanically ventilated, we have found a statistically significant correlation between Pao_2 and FRC (during oxygen breathing) (Aldredge, K., personal communication, 1971). It is therefore not surprising that in ARF, elevation of FRC by means of positive end-expiratory pressure (PEEP) is usually associated with a corresponding increase in Pao_2. However, the extent and distribution of airway closure and gas trapping in ARF remain to be established. Regional differences in compliance and resistance within the lung affect the overall emptying sequence, and these events, as well as the inability of the patient with ARF to take slow, deep breaths, mask a distinct point of beginning airway closure easily demonstrable in patients with little or no lung disease. When transpulmonary pressure and lung volume are suddenly decreased in patients with ARF (by removal of PEEP), a drastic fall in Pao_2 occurs within one minute of change in lung volume.[40] This observation is best explained by prompt alveolar closure and increase in $\dot{Q}_S/\dot{Q}_T$. Airway closure with absorption of trapped oxygen would produce more gradual atelectasis. ARF is probably associated with closure of both small airways and alveoli, depending on the nature of the acute process, presence or absence of obstructive airways disease, and integrity of the surfactant system.

Role of Surfactant in ARF

The chemistry and physiologic function of pulmonary surfactant have been the subject of several recent reviews.[42–46] The inherent instability of airspaces is normally offset by surfactant, which has the unique ability to reduce the alveolar surface tension and maintain alveolar volume at low transpulmonary pressure. With impaired surfactant function, alveolar surface tension is not reduced at low lung volumes. Progressive closure of airspaces with shunting, therefore, sets in particularly at end-expiration, when lung volume and alveolar size are least. Reinflation of closed airspaces requires high transpulmonary pressures. Greater inspiratory work is necessary to generate a sufficient opening pressure, and in the spontaneously breathing patient, this effort may lead to exhaustion, with further progression of atelectasis, pulmonary edema and respiratory failure.

Both synthesis of surfactant and the final product may be susceptible to impairment by a variety of chemical and physical stimuli. The potential role of high oxygen concentrations and mechanical ventilation as causes for surfactant depletion deserves particular attention since both are part of the treatment of the consequences of abnormal surfactant activity and ARF.

Mechanical ventilation with ambient air and normal tidal volumes does not appear to alter surfactant in the dog[47] or cause any lung damage in lambs.[48] In oxygenated isolated dog lungs there is evidence for a reversible increase in surface tension that is directly related to the size of the tidal volume and duration of ventilation, and inversely affected by the magnitude of end-expiratory pressure.[49] These data imply that restoration of normal function is dependent upon production of new surfactant by aerobic metabolic processes. There is experimental evidence, recently summarized,[45] that alveolar ventilation is sufficient to maintain surfactant metabolism in face of loss of perfusion, whereas loss of both ventilation and perfusion rapidly depletes the surfactant system. If this indeed is true for man, use of a ventilatory pattern that maintains alveolar and airway patency is important in ARF.

Ventilation of intact dogs with excessively large tidal volumes for several hours, culminating in right-sided heart failure and pulmonary edema, produced elevation in minimal surface tension of the lung extract 24 to 48 hours later.[50] Caution must be exercised when these findings are extrapolated to the clinical situation since the tidal volumes used experimentally were much larger than those commonly employed in man. However, in the presence of respiratory failure with pronounced uneven distribution of ventilation and low FRC, it is likely that some ventilated alveoli become grossly overdistended and their surfactant suffers, whereas others receive little ventilation.

Prolonged exposure to high inspired oxygen concentrations leads to depletion of extractable surfactant both in spontaneously[51] and in mechanically ventilated[47] dogs. A similar cause-effect relation was not demonstrated in the lamb.[48]

The causative role of surfactant deficiency in the production of pulmonary disease remains to be established.

Scarpelli[46] concludes that "there is no disease, including the respiratory distress syndrome, in which a primary defect of the surfactant system has been demonstrated conclusively as the etiological factor," an opinion shared by Clements.[43] It seems, then, that with the possible exception of the premature infant, surfactant deficiency is a result, not a cause, of alveolar damage. However, once surfactant deficiency has developed, the consequences in terms of lung function are serious.

3

PULMONARY EDEMA

FOR purposes of this review, "pulmonary edema" refers to the presence of a greater than normal quantity of lung water. Over the past decade it has become apparent that accumulation of water in the lung is a universal component of acute respiratory failure, even in patients without primary cardiac disease.[52] Recently, we described a clinical syndrome characterized by impaired blood gas exchange, positive water balance and radiographic changes suggestive of pulmonary edema in patients receiving prolonged artificial ventilation.[53] The frequency of respiratory failure consequent to administration of excessive colloid or salt solution to patients with trauma was recently re-emphasized.[54] Finally, lungs of patients dying with respiratory failure are characteristically heavy, often weighing 1 or even 2 kg more than normal lungs.[55-57]

Normal Physiology

Starling's dictum in relation to transcapillary exchange has been shown to apply to the lung[58-59]: net efflux or influx of water from the capillary is dependent upon the algebraic sum of the outward and inward forces. The left atrial pressure is the major intravascular force promoting egress from the capillary, and colloid osmotic pressure the primary inward force. In addition, net fluid transfer is affected by pericapillary pressures of the pulmonary interstitium. Pericapillary pressure of normal lung has been estimated to range from –7 to –16 mm of mercury,[60] thereby normally favoring egress of fluid from the vessels. However, if the pulmonary interstitial compartment becomes fluid filled and loses its negative pressure, the opposite may be true.

In the low-pressure pulmonary circuit, gravity profoundly affects the pulmonary circulation and the net hydrostatic pressure at the capillary level.[61] The division of the lung into three functional zones dependent primarily on the effective pulmonary circulatory pressures was proposed and validated by West and his associates.[62] In simple terms, at the apex of the upright lung, ventilation exceeds perfusion, since the hydrostatic pressure is inadequate to force blood that high (Zone I). At the base of the lung, perfusion exceeds ventilation (Zone III); between these zones ventilation and perfusion are relatively well matched (Zone II). A fourth zone, consisting of underperfusion in association with interstitial pulmonary edema, has been proposed.[63]

Pathologic Physiology

Although the initiating stimulus for accumulation of water in the lung varies and is not easily identified, the clinical manifestations are remarkably consistent: change in the lung ranging from localized fluffy densities to diffuse opacification on the x-ray film and evidence of progressive impairment of pulmonary gas exchange and mechanics.

The sequence of experimentally induced fluid accumulation in the lungs[19] is the same, whether caused by

massive fluid overload ("high-pressure edema") or alloxan damage to pulmonary vessels. The former is com-
parable to clinical failure of the left side of the heart or
excessive fluid administration, and the latter the experimental counterpart of the endothelial damage assumed
to occur in such diverse conditions as septic shock, pulmonary anaphylactic response and oxygen toxicity. Microscopical examination of rapidly frozen lungs showed
an orderly progression of edema, with fluid initially ac-
cumulating in the extra-alveolar interstitial connective-
tissue compartment around the large blood vessels and
airways. Alveolar-wall thickening followed, but the alveolus became fluid-filled only after the interstitial compartment was well filled. Alveolar filling occurred inde-
pendently and rapidly in individual alveoli (without
resultant air trapping) when they reached a critical configuration at which existing transpulmonary pressure
could no longer maintain stability. Recent evidence indicates that excess water first accumulates in the portions
of the alveolar septum that are rich in connective tissue.
This initial stage, although evident when electron micrographs are used, is undetectable by light microscopy.[63a]

The phenomenon of fluid accumulation occurring
initially in the interstitial space rather than the alveoli
is probably related to the observation that the pulmonary capillary is more permeable to lipid-insoluble sub-
stances (water) than the alveolar epithelium.[64] Electron
microscopy has clearly shown that the junctions of the
capillary endothelial cells are looser than those of alveolar epithelium[65] (Fig. 4). Macromolecules, such as hemoglobin, traverse the junctions of capillary endothelium
at far lower pressures than alveolar epithelium.[66] Moreover, recent experiments in isolated dog lungs have
shown that the large extra-alveolar vessels, as well as the

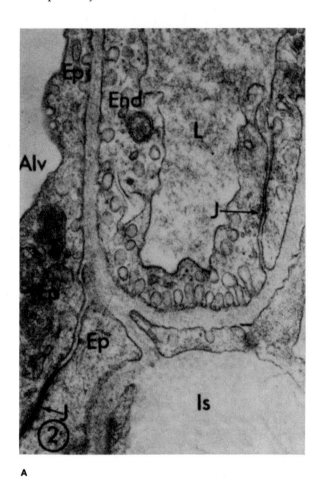

A

FIGURE 4(**A**). *See legend on page 25.*

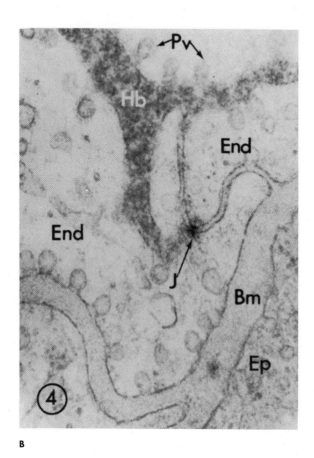

B

FIGURE 4(B).   *See legend on page 25.*

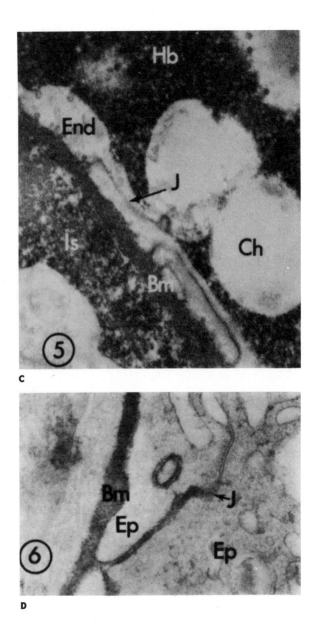

FIGURE 4(**C**) *and* (**D**). *See legend on page 25.*

capillaries, provide the portal of exit for water from the pulmonary vascular bed.[67]

In shock or sepsis, with loss of integrity of the capillary endothelium, both water and protein enter the interstitial space in the absence of increased capillary hydrostatic pressure.[68] Accumulation of edema in these circumstances is limited primarily to the dependent portions of the lung.[19] The importance of increased concentration of protein in the interstitial space is not completely apparent. If the interstitial protein concentration equilibrates with that of the vascular compartment, the colloid osmotic pressure gradient favoring intravascular reabsorption will no longer be present, thereby favoring net vascular loss of water into the lung. No abnormalities of blood gas exchange were noted in intact, spon-

---

FIGURE 4. *Electron Micrographs of the Lung, Demonstrating the Anatomic Basis for the Occurrence of Initial Extravascular Fluid Accumulation in the Interstitial Space Rather than in the Alveolus. Hemoglobin Solution (MW 64,500; Approximate Diameter 60 Å) Is Used as a Tracer* (Reproduced from Szidon et Al.[63a] with the Permission of the Publisher).

(**A**) Normal alveolar septum showing junctions between capillary endothelial cells (top arrow) and alveolar epithelial cells (bottom arrow). The junction of the endothelial cell is "loose," while that of the epithelial cell is "tight." ($\times$ 60,000.) (**B**) When the pulmonary artery is perfused at a pressure of 15 mm Hg, the tracer fills the lumen and extends along the luminal side of the cleft to, but not through, the junction of the capillary endothelium. ($\times$ 93,000.) (**C**) When the perfusion pressure is raised to 40 mm Hg, the tracer extends from the capillary lumen through the junction and into the interstitial space. ($\times$ 16,000.) (**D**) The "tight" junction of the epithelial cell prevents egress of the tracer from the interstitial space into the alveolus, despite the pulmonary artery perfusion pressure of 40 mm Hg. ($\times$ 45,000.)

Alv: alveolus, Bm: basement membrane, Ch: chylomicrons, End: capillary endothelial cell, Ep: alveolar epithelial cell, Hb: hemoglobin tracer, Is: interstitial space, L: capillary lumen, J: junction, Pv: plasmalemmal vesicles.

taneously breathing dogs subjected to normovolemic hemodilution with balanced electrolyte solution to a hematocrit of 5 per cent, despite a fall in total serum protein concentration to less than 1 g per 100 ml[69] and an increase of up to 70 per cent in lung water (measured gravimetrically). This observation emphasizes the importance of an intact pulmonary capillary bed.

As a result of the filling of alveoli, "true physiologic shunting" ("physiologic atelectasis") may occur without anatomic airspace collapse. Furthermore, since alveolar filling is the physiologically most important stage as far as gas exchange is concerned,[70] little, if any, hindrance to oxygenation or carbon dioxide elimination may be found during the early phase of pulmonary edema.* In more advanced pulmonary edema, the efficacy with which several hyperinflations of the lung (passive or active) reverse the fall in arterial oxygenation militates against alveolar-membrane thickening and diffusion limitation, and for fluid-filled alveoli, as the primary mechanism of hypoxemia. Although venoarterial shunting may be present without alveolar collapse in the presence of fluid-filled alveoli, it has been postulated that alveolar collapse per se may be followed by obligatory fluid accumulation.[1]

Measurements of Lung Water in Vivo

Since onset of clinical pulmonary edema is a late manifestation of the process of lung water accumulation, indirect methods have been used to detect it earlier.

---

* The role of interstitial pulmonary edema in impaired blood gas exchange is not established. As noted in a previous section, an increased tendency to airway closure follows interstitial edema in the isolated dog lung.[36] Interstitial edema has been suggested as the cause for basal airway closure and ventilation-perfusion ratio inequality seen in patients with cirrhosis.[71]

Among these are increase in venous admixture and P(A-aDO₂) dilution of serum electrolytes, decrease in hematocrit, weight gain and pulmonary vascular congestion on x-ray.[1] A marked fall in compliance follows severe pulmonary edema in the experimental animal[72] (Fig. 5). Unfortunately, the reproducible measurement of pulmonary compliance is difficult in patients, and at this time compliance is not a useful, sensitive clinical index of pulmonary edema.

Chinard and his associates[73] have developed an indicator-dilution technique for determining the pulmonary extravascular water content (PEVW). Two indicators (one intravascular and one which diffuses throughout the water space) are simultaneously injected into the right side of the circulation and collected from the left side. Thus, the only tissue bed traversed is the lungs. The volume of distribution of each indicator is calculated from the flow and mean transit time, and PEVW is considered the difference between the two. These technics normally detect about $\frac{1}{2}$ to $\frac{2}{3}$ of the water content of the lung as compared with gravimetric measurements.[72] However, in the presence of a greatly elevated cardiac output, they detect virtually all the lung water, whereas the percentage of water measured is decreased when low-flow states or pulmonary capillary damage exist. Although these technics are of considerable value to the investigator, their practical worth in the clinical management of acute respiratory failure remains to be established. The use of iodoantipyrine and $15\ O_2$ as diffusible indicators has been proposed and may lead to more rapid determination of pulmonary extravascular water.[74]

An increase in pulmonary extravascular water occurs in mitral stenosis, correlating with the severity of disease.[75] Advanced pulmonary emphysema is associated

27

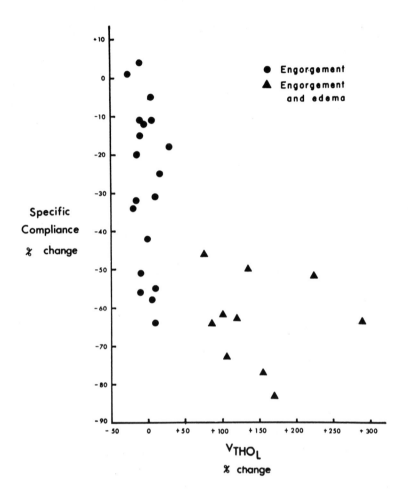

FIGURE 5. *Relation of Water Accumulation in the Lungs to Specific Compliance* (Reproduced from Levine et Al.[72] with the Permission of The American Heart Association, Inc.).

Mild pulmonary edema (engorgement) in the experimental animal is associated with a variable change in specific lung compliance. Severe pulmonary edema (engorgement and edema) always causes a marked decrease in specific lung compliance, but there is little evident relation between the degree of impairment and the severity of pulmonary edema. It is thus apparent that mild or severe edema cannot be quantitated by compliance measurements. V_{THO_L}: pulmonary extravascular water measured in vivo by the double-indicator dilution technique.

with a decrease in pulmonary extravascular water except in the presence of acute cor pulmonale, when pulmonary extravascular water rises above normal values.[76] In a group of 19 postsurgical patients, abnormally high extravascular water content was present only in those who had had a previous period of shock or sepsis.[77] There was no correlation between a positive water balance and pulmonary extravascular water, nor were any of the patients in clinical heart failure. The hypothesis was that pulmonary ischemia or sepsis had caused pulmonary capillary injury. A similar increase of pulmonary extravascular water was shown in hemorrhaged dogs who proved not to have an increase in gravimetrically determined lung water at autopsy.[78] This was considered to be an inherent methodologic error due to coronary recirculation of the indicator.

Positive Water Balance and Pulmonary Edema

On the basis of a survey of 100 consecutive patients treated with prolonged artificial ventilation, Sladen et al.[53] described a clinical syndrome characterized by a positive water balance and radiographic changes suggestive of pulmonary edema in the absence of recognizable cardiac failure or elevated central venous pressure (Table 2). There were important concomitant changes in pulmonary mechanics and gas exchange. The average weight gain at the peak of respiratory insufficiency was 2.6 kg, an amount easily overlooked unless patients are accurately weighed. Since adult patients in a catabolic state should lose 300 to 500 g in body weight daily, failure to do so is tantamount to a positive water balance. Mean daily water intake of patients in positive balance was 38 ml per kilogram (including the estimated con-

TABLE 2. *Fluid-Retention Syndrome in 100 Consecutively Ventilated Patients.**

Incidence	19%
Time to develop	4 days
Physiologic changes:	
Pulmonary edema on x-ray	
Increase in weight	2.6 kg
Increase in alveolar-arterial O_2 gradient	130 mm Hg
Fall in vital capacity	29%
Fall in effective compliance	31%
Fall in hematocrit	12%
Fall in serum sodium	6 mEq/L

* Changes associated with water retention detected in 19 of 100 consecutively ventilated patients. The data are the results of a retrospective study conducted in 1967. The mean values given were recorded during the period of maximum water retention. Water restriction and diuretic therapy reversed all these changes. Clearing of the chest x-ray did not occur concurrently in all patients.

Modified from Sladen et al.[53] with the permission of the publisher.

tribution to the respiratory water balance from humidifiers and nebulizers). Although this quantity of water is within usually accepted clinical limits, it may represent an excess in the presence of respiratory failure.

The reasons for the tendency of patients in respiratory failure to retain water are not known. Hypoalbuminemia, elevation of mean airway and intrathoracic systemic venous pressures, reduction of lymphatic flow, subclinical right-sided or left-sided heart failure, decreased renal cortical blood flow and perhaps unknown reflex or hormone mechanisms may be responsible. Decreased renal plasma flow and glomerular filtration rate secondary to hypoxemia and hypercapnia were thought to explain the tendency to pronounced water retention and edema seen in the emphysematic and bronchitic patient with ARF.[79] The role of antidiuretic hormone in this syndrome is controversial. Many disorders, including pneumonia, polyneuritis[80] and central-nervous-system disease, may be associated with the syndrome of inappropriate secretion of antidiuretic hormone.[81] Recent observations in humans have shown that IPPV causes inappropriate secretion of antidiuretic hormone.[81a] A further increase in plasma ADH level is seen with application of positive airway pressures during expiration.[82] In a study of eight mechanically ventilated patients, a changeover from intermittent positive-pressure ventilation (IPPV) to IPPV with PEEP was followed by a nearly threefold increased plasma level of antidiuretic hormone (Kumar, A., and Baratz, R., personal communication, 1972).

Prevention and Treatment of Pulmonary Edema in ARF

Constant vigilance is necessary to avoid positive water balance in patients with severe respiratory failure. Daily assessment of sodium and water balance and weighing are very helpful, although difficult to perform routinely. Unless abnormal losses are present, we prefer to limit total fluid administration in patients being mechanically ventilated to 20 to 25 ml per kilogram (1000 to 1500 ml) per 24 hours. The contribution of nebulizers to respiratory water balance must be taken into account.[53] Administration of diuretic drugs is frequently necessary to maintain water balance. Their anticipatory use is indicated when pulmonary capillary damage or overhydration is suspected.

Since capillary and venous pressure and pulmonary blood flow are greatest in the dependent portion of the lung, leakage of fluid at this site is inevitable with time. Accordingly, frequent change of position constitutes an important preventive measure against formation of regional pulmonary edema (as well as airspace closure and retention of bronchial secretions). Unless contraindications are present, the patient should be turned from side to side hourly. Turning to the semi-prone, head-up and head-down positions should be carried out several times daily for 20 to 30 minutes at a time.

The most effective immediate therapy for hypoxemia associated with pulmonary edema is to increase the inspired concentration of oxygen and to apply an appropriate pattern of ventilation. Success of subsequent measures depends on the etiology of pulmonary edema. In the absence of pulmonary capillary damage, diuretic therapy and water restriction lead to improvement of respiratory function, although radiologic changes are frequently reversed slowly.[53] In the presence of pulmonary capillary lesions with loss of capillary integrity and leakage of protein, Starling's Law no longer pertains. Even vigorous diuresis and dehydration are often ineffective. There is no evidence that a reduction in pulmonary venous pressure below normal is beneficial, but overhydration must be studiously avoided.

Although the simultaneous administration of salt-poor albumin and diuretic agent has been shown to decrease an elevated $P(\text{A-aDO}_2)$,[83] this practice usually increases intravascular volume, as does the administration of salt-poor albumin alone. Nobody has shown that albumin will selectively mobilize water from the lung; furthermore, if ARF is associated with pulmonary capillary damage, albumin will be lost into the extravascular space. The evidence is unconvincing that the combination of albumin and diuresis is of greater value in decreasing $P(\text{A-aDO}_2)$ than diuresis alone. We recommend that colloid be administered only if circulatory evidence of hypovolemia accompanies vigorous diuresis or if hypoalbuminemia is present.

If intrinsic renal function is adequate, a lack of renal response to diuretics is indicative of borderline renal blood flow despite an apparently normal blood pressure. Two factors may be responsible—namely, a contracted blood volume or marginal cardiac output. Reduced blood volume should be corrected with the appropriate intravascular colloid.

In patients with hemorrhagic or septic shock, or with drug intoxication, right atrial pressure is an unreliable guide to blood volume requirement. If whole blood, albumin or salt solutions are infused until "normal" arterial pressure and CVP have been reached in these patients, interstitial pulmonary edema and a rising $P(a\text{-}aDO_2)$ will almost invariably occur. Therefore, replacement should be considered adequate when satisfactory urinary output has been established in spite of subnormal systemic arterial or venous pressures. In contrast, a higher CVP is necessary in the presence of pulmonary embolization with right-sided failure or in atrial fibrillation. According to our experience, an element of right ventricular failure may be present after resuscitation from extensive trauma. Such patients also need a higher CVP. Mean pulmonary-artery pressure and pulmonary vascular resistance are frequently increased. One can only speculate on the reasons for these findings. Neurohumeral mechanisms, microembolization of aggregated red cells or platelets and fat emboli may all have a role. The clinical use of the Swan–Ganz catheter[84] to measure pulmonary capillary wedge (left atrial) pressures adds immeasurably to the management of pulmonary edema and estimation of left ventricular performance. Measurement of cardiac output is also helpful in guiding therapy. We consider a cardiac index of less than 4 to 5 liters per minute per m^2 inadequate in patients with ARF secondary to multiple trauma, sepsis, pneumonia, etc.

If decreased renal blood flow is secondary to inadequate cardiac output in the presence of normal or high cardiac filling pressures, it is frequently necessary to improve cardiac output by the intravenous infusion of isoproterenol or epinephrine, or occasionally by transvenous cardiac pacing. Here, too, the best end point in terms of systemic blood pressure is the return of urinary flow. A clinically applicable method of measuring distribution of renal blood flow is needed to improve care in this area.

Summary

Lung water accumulation is frequently a contributing cause of, and commonly accompanies, ARF, with serious consequences if not recognized and treated in its early stages. Its clinical recognition is based upon nonspecific symptoms and signs, and clinical quantitation is not yet feasible. Treatment should be directed along the following lines: (1) correction of hypoxemia by increasing inspired oxygen concentration. In severe ARF, artificial ventilation, including the use of positive endexpiratory pressure, should be instituted; (2) maintenance of negative water balance by diuretic therapy and water restriction. Administration of colloid is reserved for correction of hypovolemia or severe hypoproteinemia; (3) frequent change of position to prevent accumulation of fluid and airspace closure in the dependent regions of the lung; (4) meticulous care to avoid overloading the circulation with colloid and other fluids following hemorrhagic or septic shock. The widespread clinical measurement of cardiac output, left heart pressures and renal cortical and medullary blood flow should greatly increase our understanding and improve our therapy of lung water retention in ARF.

4

ASSESSMENT OF RESPIRATORY FUNCTION

ASSESSMENT of respiratory function is indispensable for the provision of adequate respiratory care at all stages of treatment: early diagnosis of pulmonary complications; estimation of the efficacy of preventive measures; establishment of criteria for institution of tracheal intubation and artificial ventilation as well as discontinuance (weaning).

Table 3 lists the respiratory-function tests that we consider useful in the management of ARF. Those used routinely are easily performed, sensitive, reproducible during both spontaneous and controlled ventilation, and generally applicable at the bedside, with a minimum of discomfort to the patient. Indications, methodology and interpretation in different types of respiratory failure have been thoroughly presented in recent textbooks and reviews.[1,7,62,85] Accordingly, only selected aspects of oxygenation, oxygen transport and ventilation that in our experience are commonly misinterpreted will be treated here.

Oxygenation and Ventilation

Interpretation of Pa_{O_2}

In the clinical setting, measurement of arterial oxygen saturation affords little physiologic information beyond

TABLE 3. *Tests for Assessing Respiratory Function in Critically Ill Patients.*

OXYGENATION

Inspired oxygen concentration (F_{IO_2})
Pao_2 on controlled & spontaneous ventilation
$P(A\text{-}aDO_2)^{1.0}$* or $P(A\text{-}aDO_2)^{0.5}$*
Hematocrit or hemoglobin concentration
Arterial oxygen content (Cao_2)†
Right-to-left shunt ($\dot{Q}_S/\dot{Q}_T$)†

VENTILATION

Tidal volume (V_T), frequency, minute ventilation ($\dot{V}_E$)
$Paco_2$
Dead-space-to-tidal volume ratio (V_D/V_T)
Carbon dioxide production ($\dot{V}co_2$)
Ventilator dead space & compression volume

VENTILATORY RESERVE & MECHANICS

Total vital capacity
1st-sec vital capacity (FEV_1)
Maximum expiratory flow rate (MEFR)
Inspiratory force
"Weaning time"
Effective compliance
Dynamic compliance†
Functional residual capacity (FRC)†
Check for ventilatory discoordination†

RELATED DIAGNOSTIC PROCEDURES

Chest x-ray & fluoroscopy†
Sputum smear & culture; antibiotic sensitivity
Body weight
Water balance
Serum & urine electrolytes
Serum protein concentration
Central venous pressure†
Mixed venous oxygen content†
Cardiac output†
Pulmonary-artery & capillary wedge pressures†

---

* Difference in alveolar-arterial oxygen tension measured during ventilation with 100 per cent & 50 per cent oxygen, respectively.

† Tests performed under special circumstances in the critically ill, unstable patient with respiratory or circulatory failure or both; facilities & technics now available for doing these more complex tests at the bedside when indicated.

an estimate of adequacy of arterial oxygenation. Additional information is provided by the Pao_2, which, when related to the inspired oxygen tension, is indicative of the efficiency of oxygenation. The physician must know not only whether arterial blood is adequately oxygenated but also the effectiveness with which oxygen is taken up in the lungs, since the latter is the most sensitive index of pulmonary complications leading to acute respiratory failure.

Efficiency of oxygen exchange is expressed by the alveolar-arterial oxygen tension difference $P(A\text{-}aDO_2)$, and the right-to-left shunt as a fraction of per cent of cardiac output $(\dot{Q}_S/\dot{Q}_T)$. In normal man at rest, $\dot{Q}_S/\dot{Q}_T$ varies from 2 to 5 per cent of the cardiac output. Values exceeding 50 per cent have been measured in patients with severe ARF and are compatible with survival only if the patient is mechanically ventilated with an inspired oxygen concentration of 80 to 100 per cent. For example, with an assumed arteriovenous oxygen content difference $(C[a\text{-}\bar{v}DO_2])$ of 6 ml per 100 ml of blood, a 50 per cent shunt would result in a Pao_2 of 40 mm of mercury in a patient breathing 100 per cent oxygen (Fig. 6).

When Pao_2 is high enough to ensure full saturation of hemoglobin (a level usually considered to be 150 mm of mercury), the shunt equation can be simplified as follows:

$$\dot{Q}_S/\dot{Q}_T = \frac{P(A\text{-}aDO_2) \cdot 0.0031}{P(A\text{-}aDO_2) \cdot 0.0031 + C(a\text{-}\bar{v}DO_2)} \times 100,$$

where 0.0031 is the factor required to convert partial pressure into oxygen content at $37^\circ C$. Precise calculation of $\dot{Q}_S/\dot{Q}_T$ thus requires measurement of mixed venous oxygen content in a pulmonary-artery sample. The Swan–Ganz balloon catheter[84] makes it possible to cathe-

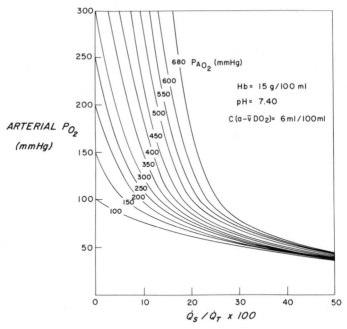

FIGURE 6. *Analogue-Computed Relation between per Cent Right-to-Left Shunt ($\dot{Q}s/\dot{Q}_T \times 100$), Pao2 and Inspired Oxygen or Alveolar Oxygen Tension (Pao2)* (Reproduced from Pontoppidan et Al. [Edited by Welch][1] with the Permission of Year Book Medical Publishers; Graph Kindly Prepared by Dr. M. A. Duvelleroy).

The P(A-aDO2) can be obtained by means of a horizontal line drawn from the ordinate (Pao2) to the appropriate Pao2 line. For example, when $\dot{Q}s/\dot{Q}_T \times 100 = 20$, and Pao2 = 680 mm of mercury, Pao$_2$ is approximately 175 mm of mercury, and P(A-aDO$_2$) = 680-175 = 505 mm of mercury. Note that below $\dot{Q}s/\dot{Q}_T$ value of 30 per cent, small changes in shunt can produce drastic alterations in Pao2, particularly when the subject is breathing high concentrations of oxygen. The curves were drawn from the shunt equation assuming a hemoglobin concentration of 15 g per 100 ml, arterial pH of 7.40, C(a-$\overline{v}$DO$_2$) of 6 ml per 100 ml, and a standard oxyhemoglobin dissociation curve.

terize the pulmonary artery of such patients whenever indicated without fluoroscopy and provides the additional advantage of allowing monitoring of both pulmonary-artery and capillary wedge pressures as guides to therapy.

Magnitude of the $P(A\text{-}aO_2)$ is determined by several factors listed in Table 4. The most obvious is the in-

TABLE 4. *Factors that Influence the Alveolar-Arterial Oxygen Tension Differences $P(A\text{-}aO_2)$.*

1. Magnitude of the right-to-left shunt ($\dot{Q}_S/\dot{Q}_T \times 100$)—i.e., % of cardiac output flowing past nonventilated alveoli
2. Inspired-oxygen concentration (any ventilation-perfusion inequality has a greater role when $<100\%$ oxygen is inspired)
3. Arteriovenous oxygen content difference ($C(a\text{-}\bar{v}DO_2)$)
4. Oxygen consumption through its effect on mixed venous oxygen content
5. Cardiac output:
   a. secondary to change in $C(a\text{-}\bar{v}DO_2)$ when oxygen consumption remains constant ($\dot{Q}_T = \dot{V}O_2/C(a\text{-}\bar{v}DO_2)$);
   b. secondary to redistribution of pulmonary blood flow.
6. Position of the arterial point of the oxygen-hemoglobin dissociation curve
7. Position of the oxygen-hemoglobin dissociation curve

spired oxygen tension. When it is high (e.g., 100 per cent oxygen), a small change in oxygen content, which is due to a right-to-left shunt, will displace the PaO_2 markedly to the left, as shown in Figure 7. The difference between PAO_2 and PaO_2 is large when the change in oxygen content is registered on the upper plateau of the oxyhemoglobin dissociation curve. If the inspired oxygen concentration is low, so that PaO_2 is not high enough to ensure full saturation, the magnitude of the $P(A\text{-}aO_2)$ will be affected by the degree of desaturation and the increasing slope of the dissociation curve. Therefore, for the same oxygen-content change (ΔCO_2^{Air}), the

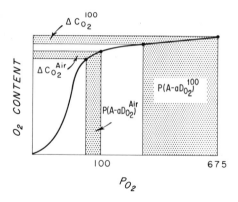

FIGURE 7. *Schematic Demonstration that a Small Fall in Arterial Oxygen Content ($\Delta Co_2{}^{100}$) during Breathing of 100 per Cent Oxygen Is Associated with a Large Increase in the Alveolar-Arterial Oxygen Tension Difference ($P[\text{A-a}Do_2]^{100}$).*

During air breathing the same change in arterial oxygen content ($\Delta Co_2{}^{\text{Air}}$) is associated with a lesser alveolar-arterial oxygen tension difference ($P[\text{A-a}Do_2]^{\text{Air}}$). The clinical implications are discussed in the text.

$P(\text{A-a}Do_2)$ will be smaller during air breathing than during oxygen breathing.

During 100 per cent oxygen breathing, the oxygen tension is the same in all ventilated alveoli (Pao_2) and is equal to barometric pressure less arterial* carbon dioxide pressure, less alveolar water-vapor pressure. Under these circumstances, the $P(\text{A-a}Do_2)$ reflects the "true physiologic" shunt arising in perfused areas of the lung that are totally without ventilation—i.e., $\dot{V}_A/\dot{Q} = 0$. Oxygen breathing thus eliminates the influence of "ventilation perfusion inequality" on the calculated right-to-left shunt[86]: any change in alveolar oxygen concentration

* Variations in alveolar carbon dioxide tension ($Paco_2$) due to ventilation perfusion inequalities are trivial as compared to the Pao_2 during oxygen breathing. The error made in assuming that $Paco_2$ equals $Paco_2$, therefore, is negligible.

can only be the result of changes in carbon dioxide, which in turn cannot rise higher than that of mixed venous blood. Thus, $P(A\text{-}aDO_2)$ is appropriately measured and simple to interpret when the inspired oxygen concentration (F_IO_2) equals 100 per cent. The time required to achieve a steady state after a change to 100 per cent oxygen breathing rarely exceeds 20 minutes and, in non-emphysematous patients, is usually less than 10 minutes.[1]

As F_IO_2 is reduced below 100 per cent, the $P(A\text{-}aDO_2)$ increasingly reflects not only the shunt effect arising from parts of the lung with a ventilation-perfusion ratio ($\dot{V}_A/\dot{Q}$) of zero ("true physiologic" shunt), but also the shunt effect of regions with ventilation-perfusion inequality ($\dot{V}_A/\dot{Q}$ finite).[86] When F_IO_2 is substantially less than 100 per cent, PaO_2 must be calculated from the more complicated alveolar gas equation,[87] and the respiratory exchange ratio must be known (or assumed to be 0.8).

As shown in Figure 6, if the $\dot{Q}_S/\dot{Q}_T$ is below 30 per cent of cardiac output, small changes are detected more readily when the PaO_2 is high (that is, 100 per cent oxygen and $PaO_2 = 680$) than when the subject is breathing ambient air ($PaO_2 = 100$).

The relation between $P(A\text{-}aDO_2)$ and F_IO_2 has practical importance for two reasons: measurement of PaO_2 during temporary ventilation with a F_IO_2 of 100 per cent is a sensitive guide to the magnitude of, and changes in, the $P(A\text{-}aDO_2)$ and $\dot{Q}_S/\dot{Q}_T$; and ARF of nonobstructive origin presents primarily as "true physiologic" shunting ($\dot{V}_A/\dot{Q} = 0$).[7,52,88] In contrast, chronic obstructive lung disease is characterized by a pronounced ventilation-perfusion inequality,[89] which, in this disease, is the primary cause of the $P(A\text{-}aDO_2)$. During oxygen breathing, the $P(A\text{-}aDO_2)$ in these patients is characteristically low[52,88] and consequently is not a useful index of changes in the pulmonary status.

$P(A\text{-}aDO_2)$ and cardiac output

The $P(A\text{-}aDO_2)$ and $\dot{Q}_S/\dot{Q}_T$ are influenced by changes in cardiac output. An increase in $P(A\text{-}aDO_2)$ of 100 mm of mercury may be the result of an increase in $C(a\text{-}\bar{v}DO_2)$ from 5 to 10 ml per 100 ml of blood as may occur with a fall in cardiac output without a concomitant change in oxygen consumption (Fig. 8); as the oxygen content of

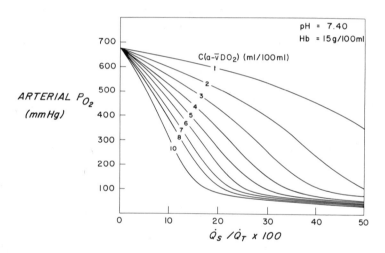

FIGURE 8. *Analogue-Computed Relation between per Cent Right-to-Left Shunt ($\dot{Q}_S/\dot{Q}_T \times 100$), Pao2 and $C(a\text{-}\bar{v}DO_2)$* (Reproduced from Pontoppidan et Al. [Edited by Welch][1] with the Permission of Year Book Medical Publishers; Graph Kindly Prepared by Dr. M. A. Duvelleroy).

Note that in the presence of a low cardiac output ($C[a\text{-}\bar{v}DO_2]$ larger than 6 to 7 ml per 100 ml), small changes in shunt, when $\dot{Q}_S/\dot{Q}_T \times 100$ is between 5 and 20 per cent, can have a striking influence on Pao2. Curves were drawn from the shunt equation assuming the same values as in Figure 2.

mixed venous blood falls, the Pao_2 decreases, the $P(A-aDO_2)$ increases, and the calculated $\dot{Q}_S/\dot{Q}_T$ is greater. Such an inverse relation of $P(A-aDO_2)$ and cardiac output was shown in a model system, verified in anesthetized patients,[90] and confirmed in patients after cardiac surgery.[91] However, other studies have shown that an increase in cardiac output was accompanied by a rise in $P(A-aDO_2)$ and $\dot{Q}_S/\dot{Q}_T$ in anesthetized patients[92] in the presence of pneumonitis,[88] mitral-valve disease[93] or cor pulmonale.[94]

A consideration of the effect of cardiac-output changes on the efficiency of oxygenation is not valid without simultaneous measurement of pulmonary-artery pressure. The effect of perfusing pressure on distribution of pulmonary blood flow is well known: if pulmonary-artery pressure and flow are augmented in relatively well ventilated regions (e.g., the upper lung regions in a sitting patient with congestive heart failure), the $\dot{Q}_S/\dot{Q}_T$ will decrease. An opposite change in $\dot{Q}_S/\dot{Q}_T$ results from redirection of flow to poorly ventilated regions (e.g., infiltrates in the upper lung in a patient in the lateral decubitus position as shown in Fig. 9). These changes in $\dot{Q}_S/\dot{Q}_T$ may be directionally the same or the opposite of those resulting from changes in $C(a-\bar{v}DO_2)$. Available data do not permit resolution of this question. The clinical implications are that a change in Pao_2 cannot be assumed to be due solely to a change in pulmonary function unless all other possible causes are accounted for.

Oxygen transport

The concept of judging adequacy of oxygenation according to the oxygen transported per minute (cardiac

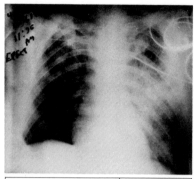

POSITION		PaO₂ (TORR)	
		s̄ PEEP	c̄ PEEP
Supine		66	97
Left Infiltrate Dependent		?	76
Left Infiltrate Nondependent		65	152

FIGURE 9. *Influence of Body Position and Positive End-expiratory Pressure on Pao2 in a Patient with Pulmonary Infiltrates in the Left Lung (Fio2 = 1)* (Reproduced from Falke et Al.[155] with the Permission of the Publishers).

Pulmonary perfusion is largely determined by gravity; the dependent portion of the lung will therefore receive the major share of perfusion. In contrast, the healthy lung will be ventilated preferentially because it is more compliant. Therefore, the highest arterial oxygen tensions are achieved when the damaged lung is nondependent (both $\dot{V}$ and $\dot{Q}$ to the dependent, healthy lung). The lowest arterial oxygen tension is achieved when the damaged lung is dependent, as most flow goes to it, increasing venous admixture. Arterial oxygen tensions are higher in all positions when PEEP is applied.

output times arterial oxygen content) requires re-examination in the light of recent observations on acutely produced, transient, normovolemic anemia. Drastic reduction of red-cell volume to an average hematocrit of 5 per cent, by replacement of blood drawn with balanced electrolyte solution in anesthetized dogs breathing spontaneously, was well tolerated and not associated with signs generally attributed to tissue hypoxia—e.g., metabolic acidosis.[69] These experiments have failed to substantiate the relevance of the oxygen-transport concept to organ function. Overall adequacy of systemic oxygenation is related to oxygen consumption of individual organs and distribution of blood flow, as well as physical characteristics of the microcirculation. The latter are critically related to viscosity (hematocrit) and the Po_2 gradient between intravascular and extravascular compartments. Unfortunately, assessment of these variables is not possible in the intact organism. However, experimental evidence suggests that the quantitative role of hemoglobin in the basal state requires renewed study.

Another reason for re-examining the classic oxygen-transport concept is recognition of adaptive factors that influence the relation between Po_2 and oxyhemoglobin saturation at a particular hydrogen ion concentration. Until recently, it was thought that alterations in the position of the oxyhemoglobin dissociation curve were rare except with changes in red-cell hydrogen ion concentration, or in the presence of carbon monoxide or methemoglobinemia. It is now clear that other factors may cause substantial, acute or chronic shifts in the dissociation curve of normal, adult hemoglobin.[95] Although clinical implications of such shifts are not clear, they merit consideration in acutely ill patients after multiple blood transfusions.[96,97]

Ventilation

Efficiency of ventilation is expressed by the arterial-end tidal P_{CO_2} difference or the ratio of dead space to tidal volume (V_D/V_T). Their measurement, correction and interpretation have recently been presented.[1,7]

Respiratory-Muscle Discoordination

Unilateral or bilateral diaphragmatic palsy, verified by fluoroscopic examination, has been observed in approximately 5 per cent of patients treated in the Respiratory Unit.[7] It was thought previously that this represented either a kind of neuromuscular derangement ("bulbar" myasthenia gravis) or direct phrenic-nerve injury during cardiac or other thoracic operations. It is

---

FIGURE 10. *Normal Respiratory Muscle Coordination* (**A**) *and Respiratory Muscle Discoordination* (**B**).

In a normal individual, excursions of chest wall and epigastrium are coordinated during both deep and quiet breathing. End-inspiration (transition from inspiratory to expiratory flow, or point-of-zero flow, second tracing from the top) occurs simultaneously with maximal chest cage and epigastrial circumference. Nonelastic belts incorporating a strain gauge were placed around the chest at the level of the fifth rib anteriorly and around the abdomen at the level of the epigastrium.

During weaning from prolonged artificial ventilation, lack of coordination of ventilatory muscle effort is common, even without any other apparent neurologic disturbance. End-inspiration occurs before the chest wall has fully expanded and coincides with a reduced circumference at the level of the epigastrium. This reduced circumference presumably reflects relaxation of the diaphragm of sufficient magnitude to reverse flow from inspiration to expiration. When the patient attempts to take a deep breath, excursions of chest wall and epigastrium increase, but the inspired volume does not change significantly. The result is labored, inefficient breathing. For further discussion, see text.

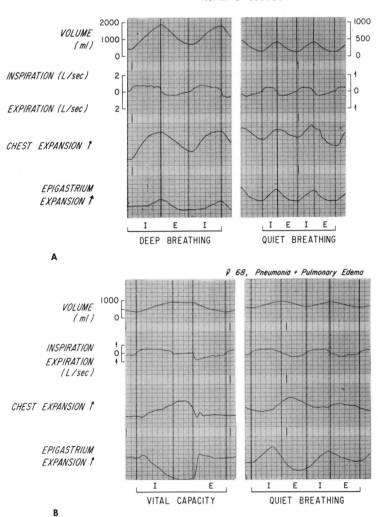

NORMAL SUBJECT

VOLUME (ml)

INSPIRATION (L/sec)

EXPIRATION (L/sec)

CHEST EXPANSION ↑

EPIGASTRIUM EXPANSION ↑

I   E   I   I E I E

DEEP BREATHING   QUIET BREATHING

A

♀ 68, Pneumonia + Pulmonary Edema

VOLUME (ml)

INSPIRATION EXPIRATION (L/sec)

CHEST EXPANSION ↑

EPIGASTRIUM EXPANSION ↑

I   E   I E I   E

VITAL CAPACITY   QUIET BREATHING

B

47

now clear that all degrees of respiratory-muscle discoordination can occur in patients with ARF, unrelated to these factors, but of sufficient magnitude to interfere with sustained, satisfactory, spontaneous ventilation and weaning from ventilator support[1] (Chiang, H., and Browne, D., personal communication, 1972). Discoordination arises from inability to synchronize the motion of the diaphragm and the muscles of the chest wall. Such a distorted respiratory pattern can easily be misinterpreted as labored breathing, but a simultaneous record of gas flow, tidal volume and chest-wall and abdominal circumference will demonstrate, for example, onset of expiration while the chest cage is still expanding (Fig. 10). Fluoroscopy may reveal rapid descent of both hemidiaphragms followed by relaxation (and expiration) during the phase when the chest is expanded. In more extreme cases, the movements of diaphragm and chest are entirely unrelated. Return to a normal synchronous pattern of ventilation occurs gradually and may delay weaning from the ventilator. The cause of discoordination is unknown.

5

PULMONARY OXYGEN TOXICITY

MOLECULAR oxygen interferes with a wide variety of cellular functions, and continuous exposure to oxygen at pressures of or near one atmosphere causes fatal pulmonary injury in all mammals thus far studied.[98]

Experiments in normal subjects exposed to oxygen at one or more atmospheres have usually been terminated with onset of subjective discomfort such as substernal distress and pain on coughing. An early effect on pulmonary function is a fall in vital capacity, which becomes more rapidly progressive after 60 hours of exposure to one atmosphere.[99] Exposure to hyperbaric oxygen at an ambient pressure of two atmospheres caused a reduction in vital capacity and pulmonary compliance after six to 11 hours,[100] but no important alteration in the pulmonary capillary bed could be discerned.[101] The role of pulmonary oxygen toxicity in patients with severe respiratory failure requiring high concentrations of inspired oxygen is still uncertain.

Clinical Data

Physiologic and morphologic changes

Two recent studies have provided data on the early pulmonary response to oxygen in the clinical setting.

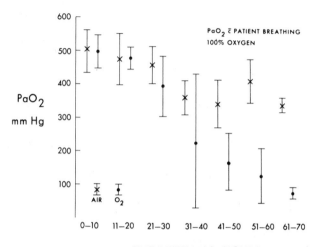

PaO₂ c̄ PATIENT BREATHING
100% OXYGEN

TIME INTERVALS - HOURS

FIGURE 11. *Effect on PaO2 of Oxygen Breathing in Patients with Normal Lungs* (Reproduced from Barber et Al.[103] with the Permission of the Publisher).

Of 10 patients who had suffered irreversible brain damage, five were mechanically ventilated with air and five with pure oxygen until death. The oxygen group demonstrated significantly greater impairment of lung function than the air group. The most sensitive indicator of impaired lung function was a decrease in arterial oxygen tension during breathing of pure oxygen. After 30 hours of ventilation, Pao2 declined more sharply in the oxygen group than in the air group. The figure shows mean values and standard deviation for sequential Pao2 in the two groups. The difference between the air and oxygen groups was significant (unpaired *t*-test) during periods from 41 to 50, 51 to 60 and 61 to 70 hours.

Singer and his co-workers[102] exposed patients mechanically ventilated after cardiovascular surgery to either 100 per cent or 50 per cent oxygen for 24 hours. At the end of this period they found no difference in lung function as determined by $\dot{Q}s/\dot{Q}T$, dead space or effective compliance between the two groups of patients. Barber et al.[103] compared the pulmonary function and morphologic changes that developed in the course of mechanical ventilation with air or oxygen in randomly selected patients with irreversible central-nervous-system disease and essentially normal lungs. The Pao_2 measured during oxygen breathing was found to be the most sensitive indicator of changes in lung function (Fig. 11). After 30 hours of ventilation this value fell sharply in the oxygen group, reaching 120 mm of mercury after 50 hours. In the air-ventilated group it declined slowly but remained above 300 mm of mercury for the duration of the study. Radiographic changes and increases of total lung weight supported these physiologic findings. In contrast, the microscopical picture was nonspecific, and no difference between the two groups was found.

Pulmonary morphologic changes after more prolonged exposure were evaluated by Nash and his co-workers,[56] who examined the lungs of 70 patients who died after prolonged artificial ventilation with various inspired concentrations of oxygen. The lungs were heavy, "beefy" and edematous. On histologic examination one could distinguish an early exudative phase characterized by congestion, intra-alveolar hemorrhage and edema. There was fibrin exudate, with the formation of prominent hyaline membranes without an associated inflammatory component. A late proliferative phase, apparent after seven to 10 days of mechanical ventilation with oxygen in concentrations of 80 to 100 per cent, was characterized by pronounced alveolar and inter-alveolar septal edema, with fibroblastic proliferation and prominent hyperplasia of the alveolar lining cells. These investigators emphasized, however, that a cause-and-effect relation between the morphologic appearance and oxygen therapy had not been documented and that many etiologic factors could have been responsible for the changes.

Role of mechanical ventilation

Of obvious concern is the role of mechanical ventilation per se in the production of the nonspecific morphologic changes. Nash and his associates[56] found that changes were unrelated to the duration of mechanical ventilation per se, but they correlated with the prolonged combined use of ventilation and high inspired oxygen concentrations. Recent animal studies throw additional light on the possible role of mechanical ventilation. In monkeys exposed to 100 per cent oxygen for up to 12 days, morphologic changes similar to those described by Nash and his co-workers,[56] including the exudative and proliferative phase, were found by Kaplan[104] and by Kapanci[105] and their colleagues. Since these animals breathed spontaneously throughout the experiment, the effects of mechanical ventilation were excluded. The role of ventilation with 80 to 100 per cent oxygen versus ventilation with air has been studied in lambs one to two weeks old.[48] Oxygen, whether breathed spontaneously or with mechanical ventilation, caused fatal pulmonary edema after two to four days. In contrast, the lungs of air-ventilated lambs did not differ from those of control animals. Similar observations in spontaneously breathing and mechanically ventilated goats exposed to air or oxygen led the authors to conclude that the term "respirator lung" is a misnomer and, again, demonstrated the lethal effects of 100 per cent oxygen regardless of the mode of ventilation.[106]

We conclude, on the basis of such data, that it is unlikely that mechanical ventilation per se could have produced the morphologic changes reported in the clinical studies of oxygen toxicity.[56,102,103] As discussed earlier, numerous conditions leading to ARF are associated with an increased tendency to closure of small airways and gas trapping. Under these circumstances, breathing of oxygen leads to absorption atelectasis,[25,32] an effect on lung function that precedes the toxic effects on cell function for hours or days. Any measure that reduces gas trapping, particularly an appropriate ventilatory pattern, should prevent this harmful effect of oxygen on lung function. The same logic can be applied to the possible effect of oxygen on surfactant function. Although evidence for damage by oxygen to surfactant is in dispute,[98] if damage for any reason occurs, an appropriate pattern of spontaneous or mechanical ventilation may minimize the catastrophic effect on alveolar patency. It seems reasonable to conclude that mechanical ventilation, instead of aggravating the toxic pulmonary manifestations of oxygen, may, in fact, prevent or delay their onset.

Modifying effect of hypoxemia and lung disease

There is no conclusive evidence that hypoxemia offers protection against pulmonary oxygen toxicity. In the dog, arterial hypoxemia produced by creation of a large anatomic $\dot{Q}_S/\dot{Q}_T$ shunt delayed, but did not prevent, the ultimate manifestations of pulmonary oxygen toxicity at two atmospheres of ambient pressure.[107] This protection was not demonstrated in similarly prepared, hypoxemic dogs exposed to one atmosphere of oxygen for two days.[108] In experimental studies the early lesion of oxygen is found in the capillary endothelium, with leakage of plasma into the interstitium and hemorrhage.[105] Because the oxygen tension of blood in pulmonary capillaries of ventilated air spaces equals that of the alveoli, one would not a priori expect arterial hypoxemia to modify any direct toxic effect on capillary integrity.

The many aspects of lung function and structure that appear to be harmed by oxygen, including the bronchial epithelium[109] and the mucus-transport system,[110] may be impaired in a variety of acute pulmonary injury and disease. Whether such a pre-existing injury renders the lung more vulnerable to the toxic effect of oxygen is not known.

Residual changes

In monkeys, the extent of residual pulmonary damage after prolonged exposure to oxygen varies with the duration of exposure.[104] Residual changes have been observed in human neonates who survived after prolonged exposure to oxygen in treatment of the respiratory-distress syndrome.[109] We have observed apparent functional reversal in two patients with severe acute respiratory failure mechanically ventilated with oxygen for more than two weeks,[1] and similar findings have been reported by others.[102,111] Systematic follow-up studies of lung function in patients after prolonged treatment with mechanical ventilation, with or without high inspired concentrations of oxygen, are needed to evaluate better the potential reversibility of pulmonary changes in ARF.

Clinical Implications

It is difficult to draw conclusions of therapeutic value from the experimental and clinical studies of pulmonary oxygen toxicity. In the assessment of patient data, one should bear in mind that interstitial and intra-alveolar edema, hemorrhage and hyaline membranes are nonspecific responses to a variety of injuries. Oxygen is only one of these, and their occurrence cannot be taken as evidence of specific oxygen effect. Overemphasis on oxygen may divert attention from factors of equal or greater importance in the pathogenesis of acute pulmonary insufficiency. Needless to say, withholding oxygen for fear of oxygen damage when the patient is severely hypoxemic may result in serious and fatal complications before the onset of pulmonary oxygen toxicity. Although man will tolerate chronic hypoxemia without ill effects, this does not predicate physiologic tolerance to acute hypoxemia, particularly in the elderly or in the patient who is acutely ill.

Current clinical practice is based on the assumption that an F_IO_2 of 50 per cent (0.5 atmosphere) or higher may produce serious changes when used for more than two days. The higher the F_IO_2, the more rapid the onset of damage.[98,112] Except in patients with chronic hypoxemia, one should select an F_IO_2 that will result in a Pao_2 in the normal range. If the $\dot{Q}_S/\dot{Q}_T$ persistently is so large (e.g., above 20 to 30 per cent—see Fig. 6) that a F_IO_2 above 50 or 60 per cent is necessary to maintain a normal Pao_2, it may be desirable to settle for a Pao_2 in the hypoxemic range. In this decision, the cardiovascular status and the patient's ability to increase oxygen transport by raising cardiac output, as well as his tolerance to hypoxemia, must be taken into account. Selection of the proper ventilatory pattern becomes especially important under these circumstances. Intermittent reduction of the inspired oxygen tension enhances tolerance to high oxygen pressures in mice.[113] If this were also true in man, taking advantage of this maneuver would be limited in patients in whom continuous high inspired oxygen concentrations are required to prevent fatal hypoxemia.

Inadvertent overdosage with oxygen and pulmonary oxygen toxicity may result from a misunderstanding of the functional characteristics of pressure preset ventilators that have a Venturi air-entrainment device.[56,111] With improved understanding[114,115] and equipment that allows precise dosage of the F_{IO_2}, this should no longer be a problem.

6

CURRENT USE OF ARTIFICIAL VENTILATION

PRECISE criteria for tracheal intubation and artificial ventilation in ARF have been difficult to define (except for their use in resuscitation). In the past, artificial ventilation was associated with serious complications and a high mortality. With the exception of pure ventilatory failure (e.g., paralytic poliomyelitis), it was the last resort when all "conservative" measures had been exhausted and death was imminent.

Recent experience has led to a fundamental change in practice. It is now accepted that artificial ventilation is often esesntial in the prevention of acute respiratory failure. Emphasis on prevention has arisen from reduction of the hazards associated with mechanical ventilation and realization that pulmonary complications usually develop insidiously over a period of several hours or days before becoming clinically manifest. Once morphologic changes have progressed sufficiently to cause obvious radiologic changes, disease is usually extensive, and ventilatory reserve severely reduced. At this point, the final stages often evolve rapidly, suggesting a sudden onset of respiratory failure. However, if respiratory function is serially evaluated, the onset of pulmonary complications can be demonstrated long before decompensation is apparent. In advanced ARF, except for cardiogenic pulmonary edema, pulmonary changes are only slowly reversible. If one delays, treatment may add to the damage owing to the need for high inspired oxygen concentrations, large tidal volumes, and high airway pressures necessary to achieve adequate gas exchange.

Work of Breathing

An elevated mechanical and metabolic cost of breathing has figured prominently in discussions of the indications for controlled ventilation,[116] the assumption being that all or part of this cost will be borne by the ventilator. In normal man at rest, work of breathing is approximately 0.5 kg-m per minute and accounts for 2 to 3 per cent of the total oxygen consumption.[117] In acute respiratory failure, the cost of breathing may rise several times over normal values. It is assumed that in the absence of obstructive airway disease, ventilatory work is primarily related to inspiration since the expiratory work is passively the result of elastic recoil of the lungs. However, in the presence of severe ARF, expiration becomes an active process.

Mechanical, controlled ventilation altered the whole-body oxygen consumption in adequately oxygenated, postoperative patients by only 7 per cent below values measured during intervals of spontaneous ventilation.[118] A larger reduction could probably be attained in patients whose respiratory work is increased owing to more marked reduction in pulmonary compliance. Examples are those with crushed chest[119] and mitral stenosis. In the latter group a change from controlled to spontaneous ventilation was associated with a 33 per cent mean increase in oxygen consumption, an oxygen cost that correlated with preoperative reduction in vital capacity from predicted, normal values.[120]

Surprisingly enough, no difference in oxygen consumption was found between controlled mechanical and spontaneous ventilation in patients recovering from ARF studied at the time of weaning from the ventilator. [1,121] On the basis of these conflicting data, the saving in oxygen cost of breathing attainable in patients with nonobstructive respiratory failure appears to be related to the clinical state at the time of study. Even if the oxygen cost of breathing is several times normal, only a small fraction of the total oxygen consumption is involved. Fever, shivering[122] and restlessness are more important factors and should also be minimized when the level of cardiac or ventilatory work is critical to survival.

Tolerance to an increased ventilatory work load is not necessarily related to the resulting increase in overall metabolic rate. Tolerance may be limited by the mechanical capacity of the muscles of respiration, which may ultimately become fatigued in response to large ventilatory demands. Factors that reduce mechanical performance and promote decompensation include respiratory-muscle hypoperfusion and hypoxemia, pronounced electrolyte and acid-base disturbances and debility. The recently recognized problem of ventilatory-muscle discoordination was discussed above.

The preceding considerations do not quite apply in patients with obstructive airway disease, in whom the oxygen cost of breathing is unusually large and expiration is an active process that cannot be assumed by mechanical ventilation.[123] Accordingly, all efforts at reducing work of breathing in patients with obstructive lung disease must be directed toward reducing the metabolic rate and carbon dioxide production by treating sepsis, fever and excessive physical activity. The high airway resistance, with its excessive work load, should be treated with bronchodilator drugs, diuretics, digitalis and corticosteroids.

Prophylactic Use of Artificial Ventilation

The value of artificial ventilation in the prevention of acute respiratory failure of noninfectious origin was first appreciated in surgical patients,[116] in whom the common occurrence of hypoxemia has long been evident.[124] Experience has shown that postoperative ven-

TABLE 5. *Guidelines for Ventilatory Support in Adults with ARF.**

DATUM	NORMAL RANGE	TRACHEAL INTUBATION & VENTILATION INDICATED
Mechanics:		
Respiratory rate	12-20	> 35
Vital capacity (ml/kg of body weight†)	65-75	< 15
FEV_1 (ml/kg of body weight†)	50-60	< 10
Inspiratory force (cm H_2O)	75-100	< 25
Oxygenation:		
Pao_2 (mm Hg)	100-75 (air)	< 70 (on mask O_2)
$P(A-aDO_2)^{1.0}$ (mm Hg‡)	25-65	>450
Ventilation:		
$Paco_2$ (mm Hg)	35-45	> 55§
V_D/V_T	0.25-0.40	>0.60

* The trend of values is of utmost importance. The numerical guidelines should obviously not be adopted to the exclusion of clinical judgment. For example, a vital capacity below 15 ml/kg may prove sufficient provided the patient can still cough "effectively," if hypoxemia is prevented, as discussed in the text, & if hypercapnia is not progressive. However, such a patient needs frequent blood gas analyses & must be closely observed in a well-equipped, adequately staffed recovery room or intensive-care unit.

† "Ideal" weight is used if weight appears grossly abnormal.

‡ After 10 min of 100 per cent oxygen.

§ Except in patients with chronic hypercapnia.

tilatory support must be considered an extension of the intraoperative management. Artificial ventilation is now widely employed in patients in whom some degree of respiratory failure is anticipated, in spite of preoperative and postoperative preventive measures, including chest physical therapy.[125,126] Susceptible patients are those in shock (regardless of cause) and those in whom recovery from operation or trauma is compromised by marked obesity, pulmonary emphysema, cardiovascular disease, muscle weakness, electrolyte imbalance or debility. The tracheas of such patients are best intubated electively before or immediately after operation with a flexible, plastic tube for controlled ventilation during the early recovery phase. Termination of mechanical ventilation and tracheal extubation can usually be accomplished within 24 to 48 hours on the basis of the physiologic principles described for weaning after prolonged ventilation.[1] These criteria are similar to those listed in Table 5 as guidelines for intubation and ventilation.

Artificial Ventilation in Primary Ventilatory Failure

Artificial ventilation was first applied to patients with primary ventilatory failure: poliomyelitis, polyneuritis, myasthenia gravis, severe tetanus and other neuromuscular disorders, chest-wall trauma with chest-wall instability and massive obesity, with or without impairment of the central regulation of breathing. The primary disturbance is a derangement of the nervous, muscular or skeletal apparatus of breathing. Pulmonary morphologic changes are secondary and invariably occur if treatment is delayed or inadequate. Physiologic criteria for intubation and ventilation that we have found useful

61

are listed in Table 5. With few exceptions, failure of lung function is heralded by a decline in vital capacity, a rise in $P(\text{A-aDO}_2)$ and elevation of respiratory rate. As the vital capacity is progressively reduced, the coughing and sighing mechanisms are impaired; sputum retention, atelectasis and pneumonitis soon ensue. Hypercapnia and respiratory acidosis are late phenomena[127] indicative of advanced ventilatory failure. Although hypoxemia may be marked in patients with severe chest injuries and flail chest wall, hypercapnia is usually not present.[128]

The Comatose Patient

A cuffed endotracheal tube must be placed in situ in deeply comatose patients to prevent aspiration of saliva, gastrointestinal contents or blood and to facilitate removal of secretions. The decision to institute artificial ventilation is based on assessment of ventilatory drive and blood gas exchange. Hypercapnia and hypoxemia both aggravate cerebral edema and are not to be tolerated in patients with acute brain injury. It is of interest, however, that hyperventilation of central origin, with marked hypocapnia secondary to cerebrospinal-fluid acidosis, is not uncommon in patients with brain damage.[129] Controlled hyperventilation to a low Paco_2, has been advocated to facilitate maintenance of a normal cerebrospinal-fluid pH.[130]

Mechanical Ventilation in ARF Secondary to Acute Pulmonary Disease and Pulmonary Edema

The largest group of patients admitted to the Massachusetts General Hospital Respiratory Unit in recent years falls in this category (see Table 1), reflecting the fact that artificial ventilation has now become accepted practice in the treatment of these patients.[9] Tracheal intubation and mechanical ventilation are increasingly used in patients with severe pneumonia (viral, bacterial or chemical), pulmonary embolism and pulmonary edema.[131]

Acute pulmonary disease is associated with an early increase in the $P(A\text{-}aDO_2)$ and ratio of dead space to tidal volume (V_D/V_T). Alveolar hyperventilation and respiratory alkalosis are characteristic of the early phase.[132,133] The ventilatory apparatus is usually intact, although weakness and fatigue secondary to the greatly increased work of breathing are eventually reflected in decreased inspiratory force. A major reduction in vital capacity invariably signifies extensive loss of pulmonary distensibility and advanced respiratory failure. The criteria for intubation and ventilation in acute pulmonary disease are the same as those for primary ventilatory failure listed in Table 5.

In the patient without an artificial airway, administration of 100 per cent oxygen requires a tight-fitting face mask and reservoir bag. The highest inspired oxygen concentration that can be reliably and continuously delivered by the standard disposable oxygen mask is 50 to 60 per cent. If the $\dot{Q}_S/\dot{Q}_T$ is so large that this oxygen concentration does not prevent arterial hypoxemia (arbitrarily taken at Pao_2 below 70 mm of mercury in Table 5), the patient should rarely, if ever, be allowed to breathe spontaneously for extended periods. (An exception may be patients acclimatized to severe hypoxemia, such as those with congenital heart disease, massive obesity or chronic pulmonary disease; in emphysema, high inspired oxygen concentrations almost invariably correct hypoxemia, and the concern is more often with avoiding their use.) When $\dot{Q}_S/\dot{Q}_T$ is large (e.g., above $\frac{1}{3}$ of the cardiac output), the increment in Pao_2 obtainable by increasing the inspired oxygen concentration from 60 to 100 per cent is small, as shown in Figure 6. Accordingly, 100 per cent oxygen affords a minimal margin of reserve in a hypoxemic patient already receiving 60 per cent oxygen. Assisted or controlled ventilation is usually followed by reduction in $\dot{Q}_S/\dot{Q}_T$ presumably by delivering the necessary opening pressure for air spaces that are fluid-filled or atelectatic. Recent experience with use of positive end-expiratory pressure indicates that this therapeutic maneuver may in some patients obviate the need for mechanical ventilation. Even when hypoxemia and hypercapnia are corrected, these patients are often tachypneic, a respiratory pattern perhaps related to the reduced pulmonary compliance.[134] Sedation (intravenous morphine or diazepam) is often required to permit synchronization with the ventilator.

Mechanical Ventilation for ARF Superimposed on Chronic Obstructive Pulmonary Disease

Indications for intubation and ventilation in this group are more stringent than those discussed above for several reasons. First of all, patients acclimated to chronic hypoxemia often tolerate extremely low levels of Pao_2 (below 40 mm of mercury) that may be fatal to the acutely ill patient without such adaptation. Secondly, ARF is often recurrent in these patients, emphasizing the special advantage of prolonged tracheal intubation over tracheostomy. Thirdly, artificial ventilation is not easily managed and in our experience is associated with a greater frequency of complications such as tension pneumothorax and a fall in cardiac output.[88] In spite of profound derangement of pulmonary mechanics and the inefficient carbon dioxide elimination, inadvertent, precipitous reduction of $Paco_2$ may follow soon after institution of mechanical ventilation. This decrease may cause cardiac arrhythmias,[135] hypotension or fatal cerebral complications, the latter presumably secondary to cerebral alkalosis, ischemia and hypoxemia.[136,137]

Finally, patients with advanced emphysema and decreased elastic recoil show less tendency for alveolar collapse and "true physiologic" shunting,[52] and do not exhibit the large reduction in FRC characteristic of patients with nonobstructive disease.[38-40] Consequently, marked reductions of vital capacity do not necessarily predispose to atelectasis. For these reasons, artificial ventilation is not indicated until all other attempts have failed to reverse hypoxemia without causing excessive hypercapnia. Such measures include treatment of infection, adequate chest physical therapy[138] and treatment of attendant bronchospasm and bronchial edema. Pulmonary extravascular water content is high in patients with acute cor pulmonale secondary to chronic lung disease with hypoxemia.[76] Left ventricular failure and edema are also common.[139,139a] Pulmonary water content decreases along with pulmonary-artery pressure and $Paco_2$ when edema is cleared by use of fluid restriction, diuretic drugs, digitalis and correction of acidemia and hypoxemia. In patients with severe hypoxemia (e.g., Pao_2 40 mm of mercury or less) a substantial rise in arterial oxygen content is attainable with a small increase in Pao_2 because the oxyhemoglobin dissociation curve is steep in this range of Pao_2. An adequate relief of hypoxemia, without attendant suppression of chemoreceptor drive and excessive hypercapnia, is the aim of "controlled oxygen therapy," which has been reported effective in the majority of patients with acute exacerbation of chronic obstructive pulmonary disease.[140-143]

Bronchial Asthma

The asthmatic person differs from the patient with emphysema by having an unimpaired respiratory response to carbon dioxide. The $Paco_2$ in severe asthma is characteristically low, and the rise to normal or hypercapnic levels a late phenomenon[144] signifying severe fatigue and decompensation. In a group of patients with severe bronchial asthma, hypercapnia did not develop until the first-second vital capacity (FEV_1) had fallen below 15 per cent of the predicted normal; the average $Paco_2$ elevation was only 10 mm of mercury. In contrast, hypoxemia was present even in mild attacks of asthma and became severe as the attack progressed.[144] Such patients must be continuously observed, and facilities for prompt intubation and assisted ventilation must be at hand. If progressive hypercapnia and exhaustion develop despite treatment with high-humidity oxygen, bronchodilator drugs and corticosteroids, nasotracheal intubation and assisted ventilation are indicated. Heavy sedation (diazepam, morphine) and occasionally paralysis (by means of *d*-tubocurarine) are required to facilitate adequate artificial ventilation.

Bronchial lavage

General anesthesia may provide some bronchodilatation, but it improves neither pulmonary mechanics nor gas exchange[145] and is rarely used in status asthmaticus. Persistence of symptoms is partly a consequence of mechanical obstruction by mucus plugs, and bronchial lavage under general anesthesia has been shown to be of special value when severe asthma is refractory to more conservative forms of therapy.[146-149] The procedure requires considerable expertise. It is best performed through a cuffed endotracheal tube (with bronchoscopes, large leaks are invariably present, particularly when airway pressures are high during positive-pressure breathing). It is important that high concentrations of oxygen be employed throughout, for the process of lavage may temporarily impair oxygenation.[147]

7

EFFECT OF MECHANICAL VENTILATION AND AIRWAY PRESSURES ON CIRCULATION

THE ventilatory pattern is defined by: the inspiratory and expiratory flow rates and pressures, including plateaus (periods of zero flow at end-inspiration or expiration); tidal volume; duration of inspiration and expiration and frequency and magnitude of hyperinflations. The optimal pattern for artificial ventilation varies from patient to patient according to the nature of the underlying disease. Ventilators must therefore provide means for altering ventilatory patterns over a wide range, features now incorporated in most volume-preset ventilators. Although the need for adequate carbon dioxide removal must be considered in the selection of appropriate ventilator settings, the larger consideration must be paid to the short-term and long-term effects of ventilator patterns on pulmonary mechanics and gas distribution and on arterial oxygenation and circulation.

Systemic Circulation

Most studies on the effect of mechanical ventilation on the circulation and blood gas exchange have been limited to a brief interval, the end point being an acute steady state. The basic reference involving normal subjects is that of Cournand and his associates,[150] who documented the importance of a pressure wave pattern producing a low mean airway pressure ("Type 3"), thereby avoiding circulatory depression. In long-term artificial ventilation, compensatory reactions such as increased venomotor tone, and change in circulating blood volume, may develop and alter the circulatory response when subsequent comparisons of artificial and spontaneous ventilation are made. Moreover, data on circulatory responses obtained in patients with normal lungs do not necessarily apply to conditions associated with respiratory failure with abnormal pulmonary mechanics, blood volume or cardiac function.[40,88]

Circulatory tolerance to mechanical ventilation depends largely on the extent to which airway pressures are transmitted to the intrathoracic blood vessels. The stiffer the chest wall, the more compliant the lung, the greater the increase in lung volume and the longer the lung is held in the inflated state, the more profound the effect on the systemic circulation. Restoration of the pressure gradient from the extrathoracic to the intrathoracic veins by a compensatory rise in peripheral venous tone is necessary for maintenance of blood flow.[151] Patients with sympathetic dysfunction (e.g., idiopathic polyneuritis, cervical-cord transection, chronic intake of antihypertensive and ganglion-blocking medication) and a low blood volume[152] may not be able to increase venous tone when IPPV is instituted. In such patients administration of plasma expander helps to restore adequate venous return and augment cardiac output (Fig. 12).

In postoperative thoracic surgical patients studied after approximately 24 hours of artificial ventilation, a

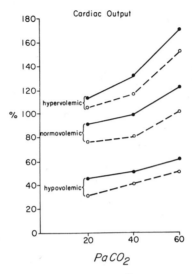

FIGURE 12. *Effect of Changes in Ventilatory Pattern on Cardiac Output in Hypovolemic and Hypervolemic Animals* (Reproduced from Morgan et Al.[152] with the Permission of the Publisher).

Changes in cardiac output in dogs (measured by an ultrasonic flow transducer implanted on the descending thoracic aorta) with alteration in ventilatory pattern and $Paco_2$. Solid lines indicate low level of ventilation, i.e., peak airway pressure 10 cm H_2O, inspiratory:expiratory time ratio 1:2. Dashed lines indicate high level of ventilation, i.e., peak airway pressure 30 cm H_2O, inspiratory:expiratory time ratio 2:1. In the hypervolemic animal, even a combination of inappropriate ventilatory pattern and massive hyperventilation did not depress cardiac output below control. In contrast, the intolerance of the hypovolemic animal to mechanical ventilation is clearly shown.

23 per cent increase in cardiac index was found upon changing from controlled to spontaneous ventilation. The concomitant rise in oxygen consumption was only 8 per cent. Therefore, the lower cardiac index during controlled ventilation could not be attributed solely to

reduced energy requirements as compared with spontaneous breathing.[118]

In the course of artificial ventilation, a change in ventilatory pattern affects the cardiac output less than during transition from spontaneous to controlled ventilation or vice versa. For instance, reduction in mean airway pressure by the addition of a negative-pressure phase during expiration did not change cardiac output in the studies referred to above[118] or in a group of anesthetized patients.[153] Even a very large increase in tidal volume and mean airway pressure (respiratory frequency constant at 20 per minute) in patients with pneumonia and pulmonary edema was not accompanied by a fall in cardiac output.[88] An important exception was found in patients with severe emphysema, in whom these large increases in tidal volume led to a marked decline in cardiac output. This was probably secondary to air trapping at end-expiration and inadequate emptying of the lungs, with further impairment of venous return. Such air trapping is common when the airway resistance is high and the elastic recoil of the lung low. Other contributing factors may have been large changes in pleural pressure after increased airway pressures in patients with compliant lungs and noncompliant chest wall and an increase in pulmonary vascular resistance, aggravating subclinical failure of the right side of the heart.

The largest increase in mean airway pressure is found during ventilation with PEEP, recently widely used in patients with grave, acute respiratory failure and hypoxemia. Here, the circulatory response is variable. In a study in dogs, in which severe ARF was produced by intravenous oleic acid injection, PEEP caused a large fall in cardiac index, while improving compliance and Pao_2.[154] Presumably, these dogs were acutely hypovo-

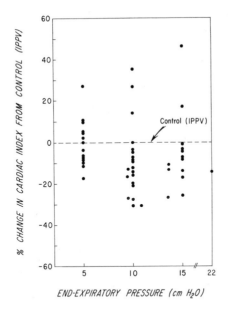

FIGURE 13. *Changes in Cardiac Output with Different Levels of PEEP in Patients with ARF.*

Note the large variation in hemodynamic response. The change in cardiac output caused by even a high level of end-expiratory pressure is unpredictable in any given individual and is dependent upon factors including blood volume, underlying pulmonary pathology and competence of the autonomic nervous system. On the average, however, only minor change in cardiac output occurs with 5 cm H2O end-expiratory pressure, whereas a mean decrease of approximately 15 to 20 per cent (compared with IPPV) occurs when 10 to 15 cm H2O PEEP is present.

This figure includes data from three studies (refs. 39, 40, 155). In the last two of these, the experimental data are obtained after removal of end-expiratory pressure in patients subjected to PEEP for several hours or days. The "control" state was thus IPPV with PEEP. If true circulatory adaptation occurs during this period, it may be necessary to exercise caution in drawing conclusions regarding the expected hemodynamic response when first applying PEEP.

lemic as a result of the massive pulmonary edema produced by oleic acid injection. The circulatory response
in patients is, as might be expected, less predictable (Fig.
13). IPPV with an end-expiratory pressure of 5 cm of
water failed to alter cardiac index in five patients
studied.[39] In another group of 10 patients, the hemodynamic response to four different levels of plateau expiratory pressure (0, 5, 10 and 15 cm of water) was varied,
with a fall in cardiac index in some and a rise in others,
but without noteworthy change in mean cardiac index,
even at the highest level.[155] In another study of eight patients exposed to expiratory flow impedance, reapplication of an average end-expiratory pressure of 13 cm,
after a 30-minute interval of ventilation with zero expiratory pressure (IPPV), caused a 20 per cent reduction
in cardiac index without change in arterial blood pressure.[40] Mean airway pressure rose from 11 to 23 cm of
water. In both studies the "control" state was IPPV with
PEEP. The relative hypervolemia, secondary to reduction in mean airway pressure during the interval of
IPPV, probably increased hemodynamic driving pressure, elevating the cardiac output above values found
with IPPV plus PEEP. (In the dog a compensatory increase in blood volume was required for tolerance of increased mean airway pressure during artificial ventilation.[152]) It is noteworthy that the cardiac index during
ventilation with PEEP was normal, or above normal, in
seven of the eight patients.

In both animals and anesthetized patients, change in
$Paco_2$ has been found to be an important regulator of
the circulatory response to artificial ventilation.[152,153]
When changes were induced in $Paco_2$ during constant
volume ventilation, there was a positive correlation between $Paco_2$ and cardiac output.[153] In contrast, in a

group of conscious patients with ARF, a large reduction in $Paco_2$ associated with an increased minute ventilation did not alter cardiac output.[88] Similarly, in normal, conscious human subjects decreasing $Paco_2$ below normal during controlled ventilation did not change cardiac index, but an increase above normal was followed by proportional rises in cardiac output.[156]

In summary, clinical experience supported by studies in patients with ARF suggests that the systemic circulatory response to IPPV and PEEP is not as predictable as demonstrated in laboratory animals or found in normal human volunteers. A transient reduction in cardiac output may be expected when artificial ventilation is first initiated, and a rise when it is terminated. Once circulatory adjustment to artificial ventilation has occurred, variations in ventilatory pattern, even with large changes in mean airway pressure, are generally well tolerated except in patients with advanced emphysema, diminished blood volume or impaired sympathetic nervous activity.

Pulmonary Vascular Response to Artificial Ventilation

The pulmonary vascular resistance in excised dog lungs is primarily volume dependent, being lowest at 50 per cent of maximal lung volume.[157] The least total resistance obtains presumably at FRC. The resistance to flow in the small, interalveolar vessels (below 30 μ in diameter) that are exposed to alveolar pressure increases with rising lung volume. The larger vessels (above 100 μ in diameter) are affected by interstitial pressure, and their resistance falls as lung volume increases.[158] When mechanical ventilation is instituted, one would therefore expect the pulmonary vascular resistance to change with major changes in lung volume. If the initial lung volume is below normal, a decrease in pulmonary vascular resistance may follow initiation of mechanical ventilation. This may explain the fall in resistance when changing from spontaneous to controlled ventilation as observed in a series of postoperative thoracic surgical patients.[118] If the initial lung volume is close to normal FRC or above, further elevation of lung volume may be associated with an increase in pulmonary vascular resistance.

Many different kinds of stimuli increase pulmonary vascular resistance.[54,159] Among these are acidosis, hypoxemia, pulmonary ischemia after pulmonary-artery ligation and hemorrhagic shock, pulmonary edema, red-cell or platelet emboli in septic shock or after multiple blood transfusions and a variety of neurohumoral mechanisms. Data on the influence of these factors in man are not available, since we lack information of the pulmonary vascular response in ARF. They may be responsible for the common observation of an increased pulmonary vascular resistance in ARF. Under these circumstances, right atrial pressure reflects right ventricular performance rather than adequacy of volume replacement.

8

VENTILATORY PATTERN AND GAS EXCHANGE

Oxygenation

Tidal volume and $P(\text{A-aDO}_2)$

The ventilatory pattern profoundly affects the efficiency of oxygenation by affecting the lung volume. Progressive alveolar or airway closure with nonventilation of perfused alveoli most probably explains the increase in $P(\text{A-aDO}_2)$ observed during prolonged constant-volume ventilation using small tidal volumes in the absence of intermittent hyperinflations.[160–162] Passive hyperinflations restored normal compliance and blood gas exchange. Many observers have since failed to demonstrate progressive hypoxemia and shunting in anesthetized animals and patients during constant-volume ventilation.[163] However, experimental conditions differed considerably from study to study. Moreover, values for resting lung volume and its relation to closing volume, now recognized as being of critical importance to a discussion of airspace collapse and hypoxemia, have not as a rule been reported. In one study in which FRC was measured, preoperative values were below normal, and the patients had cardiopulmonary disease.[41]

In addition to the magnitude of the tidal volume, the

duration of controlled ventilation is an important determinant of change in $P(A\text{-}aDO_2)$. A group of anesthetized patients without demonstrable lung disease were carried on controlled ventilation for 24 hours at constant tidal volumes varying from patient to patient.[164] Passive hyperinflations at regular intervals were incorporated. The $P(A\text{-}aDO_2)$ was unchanged with tidal volumes of 7 ml per kilogram of body weight. However, larger tidal volumes were associated with a reduction in $P(A\text{-}aDO_2)$, and smaller volumes with its rise.

Extensive clinical experience in conscious patients indicates that volumes of 7 ml per kilogram, even with half-hourly manually applied deep breathing provided around the clock, is poorly tolerated. Patients complain of dyspnea and inadequate chest expansion even though Pao_2 and $Paco_2$ are normal. Consequently, larger tidal volumes (10 to 15 ml per kilogram) are preferable, having been used in several thousand ventilated patients with no evidence of development of pulmonary damage. Excessive hypocapnia is easily corrected by introduction of mechanical dead space.[165]

Ventilators that incorporate more frequent (every two to 10 minutes) automatic hyperinflations to a preset pressure or volume may prevent progressive atelectasis and obviate the need for large tidal volumes and mechanical dead space. However, patient tolerance and the long-term effect of such ventilatory patterns on circulation and pulmonary function are not known.

Flow pattern during inspiration also affects the efficiency of gas exchange. An inspiratory plateau pressure causes an increase in Pao_2 in the dog ventilated with air,[166] and a decrease in the V_D/V_T and $\dot{Q}_S/\dot{Q}_T$.[167]

Use of positive expiratory pressure during spontaneous and mechanical ventilation

Previously in this review we pointed out the major importance to the efficiency of oxygenation of the resting lung volume, in turn influenced by the level of end-expiratory pressure. Application of continuous positive airway pressure of 2 to 5 cm of water by face mask during spontaneous breathing—continuous positive-pressure breathing (CPPB)—was advocated many years ago by Barach[168] as an effective supplement to oxygen therapy in patients with acute pulmonary edema secondary to left ventricular failure or inhalation of toxic gases. The rationale for this treatment was its effect in decreasing venous return and in exerting pressure on the pulmonary capillaries, thereby reducing egress of fluid. Expiratory or continuous positive pressure was also advocated to reduce tracheobronchial secretions and pulmonary edema in spontaneously breathing patients after tracheotomy for long standing laryngeal obstruction (Fig. 14). Finally, CPPB was recommended by Barach in patients with obstructive pulmonary disease to maintain airway patency during expiration. After the recent demonstration of the value of adding PEEP to the mechanically ventilated patient with severe hypoxemia, there has been renewed interest in the use of CPPB during spontaneous breathing in ARF. Thus, application of CPPB during spontaneous breathing, with either an endotracheal tube or a head-enclosing chamber, was recently found highly effective in correcting the hypoxemia and low compliance of the respiratory-distress syndrome of the newborn.[169] Our experience has been that in selected intubated patients with severe acute respiratory failure, CPPB with pressures up to 10 cm of water

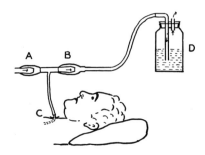

FIGURE 14. *Positive End-expiratory Pressure During Spontaneous Ventilation, also Referred to as Continuous Positive-pressure Breathing (CPPB)* (Reproduced from Barach, AL: Physiologic Therapy in Respiratory Disease. Second edition. Philadelphia, JB Lippincott Company, 1948, with the Permission of the Publisher).

CPPB was first used more than 25 years ago by Dr. Alvan L. Barach, as illustrated in this figure. Higher levels of positive end-expiratory pressure, using a modified, valveless system, are now widely used to increase lung volume and reduce shunting and hypoxemia in infant and adult patients with many different forms of acute respiratory failure.

Unidirectional valves (A and B) are not needed when the inspired gas mixture is delivered to the tracheotomy (C) at high flows or if a capacitance is introduced in the inspiratory line. A 5- or 10-liter anesthesia rebreathing bag serves as a satisfactory capacitance for the average adult. Widebore tube (D) dips under water surface for adjustable level of PEEP.

(using a modified, valveless system) may obviate the need for, and permit weaning from, mechanical ventilation that would otherwise not be tolerated owing to excessive hypoxemia.

Frumin and his associates[170] demonstrated an increase in arterial oxygenation with positive end-expiratory pressure in anesthetized, mechanically ventilated patients. This technic has recently been shown to be valuable in the treatment of a large $P(A\text{-}aDO_2)$ and hypoxemia in patients with severe ARF not responding to

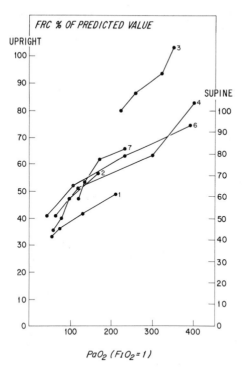

FIGURE 15. *Effect of End-expiratory Pressure on FRC and* Pao2 (Reproduced from Falke et Al.[155] with the Permission of the Publisher).

Patients with ARF were mechanically ventilated with end-expiratory pressures of 0(IPPV), 5, 10 and 15 cm H_2O in random order. There was correlation between FRC and Pao2. Each lowest point represents the relationship during IPPV, the next at 5 cm PEEP, etc. Values for predicted FRC are from ref. 4.

other means of therapy.[39,40,171] The degree of increase in Pao2 with end-expiratory pressure is related to the resulting increase in lung volume (Fig. 15). A mean increase in Pao2 of 68 mm of mercury and FRC of 0.35 liter was produced by PEEP of 5 cm of water.[39] With a pressure of 13 cm of water in another study, the corresponding changes were 179 mm of mercury and 1.18

EFFECT OF CPPV ON ARTERIAL OXYGEN TENSION

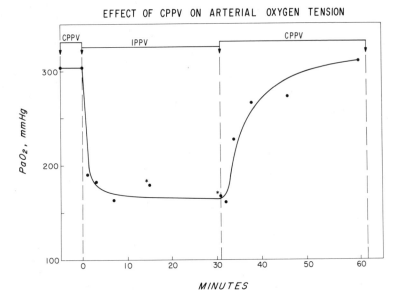

FIGURE 16. *Time Sequence of PaO2 Change with Alteration of Ventilation Pattern in Eight Patients with Severe ARF* (Reproduced from Kumar et Al.[40] with the Permission of the Publisher).

The patients had required PEEP (referred to as CPPV in the figure) with 50 per cent oxygen or less for four to 16 days before the study. Arterial samples were drawn one, three, seven, 15 and 31 minutes after change in ventilation pattern. The mean PaO2 with PEEP was 304 mm of mercury. After a change to IPPV, it fell 129 mm of mercury within one minute, with a further fall of 32 mm of mercury over the next 30 minutes. Open circles represent mean values of only six patients. (In one patient a large fall in PaO2 required reapplication of PEEP after six minutes; a second value was not available owing to clotting of the blood sample.) On reapplication of PEEP, the PaO2 rose gradually to its initial value.

liters, respectively.[40] The stiffer the lung, the less the increase in lung volume for a given level of PEEP. Accordingly, a larger rise in PaO2 can be expected in patients with both low lung volumes and relatively high pulmonary compliance.[155] Unfortunately, this is not a frequent combination clinically.

The means by which PEEP (or CPPB) relieves hypoxemia has not been established. There are several possibilities. The first consists of prevention of alveolar collapse or airway closure (Fig. 2). Most probably, PEEP is fully transmitted to the small airways and alveoli, preventing their closure and shunting during the expiratory phase. That prevention of closure of gas exchanging airspaces is entailed is indicated by the initial rapid fall in arterial oxygen tension after changeover to ventilation with *zero* end-expiratory pressure[40] (Fig. 16). The subsequent, more gradual, progressive fall in Pao_2 may be evidence for prior gas trapping that set in when expiratory pressure was lowered. As the trapped oxygen is absorbed, oxygen tension in capillary blood falls toward mixed venous levels. Other possible means of relieving hypoxemia include flattening of alveolar fluid against alveolar walls, decreasing diffusion distance,[18] decreasing effective circulating blood volume (internal phlebotomy), increasing the pressure gradient between alveolar and pulmonary capillary pressure, thereby converting "Zone 3" to "Zone 2"[172,173] and decreasing the gradient between the intravascular and extravascular pressures of the perialveolar vessels, resulting in a net influx of water into the capillaries from the alveoli and interstitial space.[168] There is no evidence, however, that PEEP reduces the total pulmonary water content.

Criteria that should be met before institution of PEEP include the following[40]: inability to maintain a Pao_2 of 70 mm of mercury with an inspired oxygen concentration of 50 per cent or more during IPPV; failure of other therapeutic measures to reduce the $\dot{Q}_S/\dot{Q}_T$ (e.g., treatment of cardiac failure, prevention or correction of fluid overload, postural change, therapy for pneumonia, atelectasis and retention of secretions); and adequate blood volume as indicated by the circulatory response to PEEP.

The level of end-expiratory pressure is guided by the response of the Pa_{O_2}, magnitude of $\dot{Q}_S/\dot{Q}_T$, lung volume and pulmonary compliance. Values as high as 20 cm of water may be required in mechanically ventilated patients before an appreciable increase in Pa_{O_2} results, when respiratory failure is pronounced. In the face of a low pulmonary compliance, PEEP with standard ranges of tidal volume results in excessively high inspiratory airway pressures. We then prefer gradual reduction of tidal volume while observing the effect on Pa_{O_2}. Maintenance of adequate minute ventilation may require an increase in ventilatory rate.

Although retardation of expiratory flow by constriction of the exhalation port can be used to generate PEEP,[40] there is no evidence that this is more effective than use of expiratory plateau pressure, and it may be more hazardous by allowing buildup of high airway pressures.[40] A simple and safe method of producing plateaus of positive airway pressures during expiration consists of immersion beneath a water surface of a wide-bore tube originating from the exhalation port of the ventilator, or from the T-piece during spontaneous breathing.[168] Attachments to ventilators for producing adjustable expiratory plateau pressure are available commercially.

The response to a trial of PEEP is not predictable. In a minority of patients PEEP fails to improve or worsens Pa_{O_2}. In rare cases this may be explained by the presence of a right-to-left intracardiac shunt,[40] but as a rule the cause is not apparent. It is possible that, under certain clinical circumstances, an increase in mean airway pressure and lung volume will cause extensive redistribution of pulmonary blood flow to nonventilated regions, thus augmenting intrapulmonary shunt flow and venous admixture.

Despite an increase in arterial oxygen content seen with PEEP in most patients with large shunts, the overall oxygen transport may fall if the depression of cardiac output is marked. The physiologic importance of such a fall in oxygen transport, however, is unknown. It must be viewed in the perspective of reversal of arterial hypoxemia, improved tissue Po_2 level, and a reduced hazard of pulmonary oxygen toxicity when sustained use of high inspired oxygen concentrations is no longer required to maintain adequate Po_2 levels. It is, of course, also possible that in some patients a higher cardiac output without use of PEEP is a physiologic response to hypoxemia. A fall with PEEP may merely reflect improved Pao_2 levels.

Use of PEEP may be associated with an increased rate of complications such as pressure trauma (subcutaneous or mediastinal emphysema and tension pneumothorax). It is likely that complications are related more to the type and degree of pulmonary disease than to the ventilatory pattern. Prospective and retrospective analysis of our experience at the Massachusetts General Hospital showed a similar incidence of pressure trauma in patients receiving IPPV or IPPV with PEEP. Although oxygenation is improved and can be maintained at normal levels in many patients, *PEEP does not preclude a fatal outcome from other systemic disturbances or progression of the pulmonary disease and destruction.*

Carbon Dioxide Elimination

The minute ventilation ($\dot{V}_E$) required to maintain a given $Paco_2$ is dictated by the magnitude of the carbon dioxide production and the efficiency of ventilation in removing carbon dioxide from the blood (V_D/V_T). Although both variables are reasonably predictable in patients with ventilatory failure and normal lungs,[174] predictability of carbon dioxide production and the V_D/V_T does not obtain in the presence of acute or chronic lung disease. Under these circumstances, both are usually elevated, and the average minute ventilatory requirement for maintenance of a normal $Paco_2$ is 50 per cent above the predicted.[52] V_D/V_T is influenced more by pulmonary-artery pressure[175] (with the attendant alteration in the distribution of pulmonary blood flow) than by the pattern of ventilation. Thus, V_D/V_T is largely independent of the magnitude of tidal volume, although a slight reduction is seen when the tidal volume is increased.[38]

Use of PEEP in the dog without lung dysfunction has been associated with an increase in V_D/V_T.[176] In patients with ARF, the use of PEEP without alteration of the tidal volume failed to change the V_D/V_T, indicating that no major redistribution of pulmonary blood flow took place.[40] In the seated normal subject, the normally occurring vertical gradients of $\dot{V}_A/\dot{Q}$ from apex to base were only minimally altered when IPPV with PEEP replaced spontaneous breathing; however, there was a slight trend to more even distribution of ventilation (and presumably smaller V_D/V_T) with PEEP.[177] Similar data are not available for patients with ARF, but redistribution of ventilation can be expected if airspace closure is eliminated as a result of increase in lung volume.

Reassessment of patterns of artificial ventilation is indicated in the light of improved understanding of airway closure and distribution of gas and blood flow in normal subjects and in respiratory failure, and of the physiologic effects of varying ventilatory patterns. Ventilator settings must be tailored to the individual patient on the basis of efficiency of blood gas exchange, and the effect on compliance, lung volume and circulation.

9

TRACHEAL INTUBATION
AND TRACHEOSTOMY

OVER the last decade, concepts in the use of artificial airways in the management of acute respiratory insufficiency have undergone major change. Prolonged tracheal intubation has received widespread acceptance, and the need for tracheostomy has, in many cases, been obviated.[178-181] For acute respiratory obstruction, the speed and ease with which intubation can be accomplished has made it the technic of choice. Emergency tracheostomy, an operation fraught with hazards, has thus become justifiable only when tracheal intubation is not possible.[182]

There is little to choose between prolonged oral intubation and nasotracheal intubation. The nasal tubes are better tolerated in conscious unsedated patients, permit closure of the mouth, and are more easily anchored. However, tube size is limited by the nostrils and turbinates. Being both longer and narrower, the tubes also provide greater resistance to gas flow, are harder to keep patent and are more apt to kink. Choice is largely dictated by the competence and interest of the staff. At the Massachusetts General Hospital, most patients after cardiac surgery are managed with orotracheal tubes, whereas most of the patients in the Respiratory Unit are managed with nasotracheal tubes.

With prolonged intubation, sudden occlusion by plugging or kinking is a major hazard, especially in the presence of lower airway bleeding. Obstruction by secretions is not always preventable, even when humidification is adequate. Facilities for prompt replacement of tracheal tubes, therefore, should always be available at the bedside.

Laryngeal Injury After Prolonged Tracheal Intubation

Ulceration of the larynx is the fundamental lesion that follows endotracheal intubation.[183,184] When intubation has been brief, the erosion is usually superficial and heals readily. Deeper and more extensive ulceration may, however, occasionally occur. In cases in which intubation has been prolonged, severe damage presenting as hoarseness, difficulty with swallowing, impaired laryngeal activity and varying degrees of respiratory obstruction has been found in up to 14 per cent of patients.[182, 184-188] The sites most commonly affected are posterior at the level of the arytenoids and in the subglottic region. Edema is invariably present, being proportional to the extent and depth of ulceration, but its effect on the airway is influenced by both its degree of severity and its location. Supraglottic edema, a frequent post-intubation complication, seldom poses any serious threat to the airway unless extensive. In the subglottic region, however, outward expansion is limited by the cricoid cartilage, and even minimal swelling can impinge upon the laryngeal lumen sufficiently to cause stridor and compromise airflow.

Granulation may follow ulceration. Usually, regression is spontaneous, without any need for active treatment unless respiratory obstruction threatens. With healing of laryngeal ulcers, laryngeotracheal membranes and vocal-cord adhesions may form. Either may cause respiratory obstruction, but both are easily amenable to corrective surgery. Healing of deeper ulcers is of greater moment. This may subsequently cause fibrotic stenosis at the subglottic level or immobilization of one or both cords from fibrosis around the cricoarytenoid joint and result in serious respiratory obstruction.[184] Surgical correction may be difficult, involving a series of complex operations.

Etiology

Laryngeal damage after prolonged tracheal intubation is primarily the consequence of pressure necrosis. The tube, by virtue of its curve, normally lies posteriorly on the glottis in apposition with the relatively firm vocal processes of the arytenoids—hence the predilection for arytenoid damage. A snug fit through the larynx enhances this effect and greatly increases the frequency of serious laryngeal damage.[182–184,189,190] This is especially likely to occur when a relatively large tube is used or when swelling is present as in children with laryngeal edema and croup.[191]

Trauma to the larynx during intubation or later as a result of movements of either the head or the tube also aggravates laryngeal damage.[188] This can be minimized by gentle intubation and sedation when patients are restless or coughing against the tube.

Irritation can occur in response to noxious materials within the tubular substance.[192,193] Rubber has a variable composition and may cause tissue damage, as may endotracheal tubes sterilized with ethylene oxide. The outward diffusing gas reacts with tissue fluids to form ethylene glycol and ethylene chlorohydrin, two toxic and irritant compounds. Damage is avoided if materials sterilized in this fashion are adequately aerated before use.[194-196]

The many complications cited make it impossible to define precisely a "safe period" for prolonged intubation. With these provocative influences minimized, however, we use endotracheal tubes in adults for up to eight days, and in children and infants for up to three weeks. Despite the possibility of regional damage, we have found prolonged tracheal intubation to be a safe procedure if carefully practiced and of special value when short-term postoperative ventilatory support is required.

Tracheal Deformity After Tracheostomy for Artificial Ventilation

Prevalance

The exact prevalence of symptomatic tracheal damage is unknown. In the past, it has been reported to occur in less than 2 per cent of cases. Recently, however, recognition of this problem has become more frequent, and the reported figure has ranged up to 20 per cent among patients receiving ventilatory support.[197] At the Massachusetts General Hospital, 57 patients with symptomatic tracheal stenosis and malacia have been treated with surgical resection and reconstruction since 1962. In 17 the lesions had developed during treatment at this hospital, representing approximately 1 per cent of the patients on mechanical ventilation for more than 24 hours.

The clinical syndrome consists essentially of upper-airway obstruction after a period of mechanical ventilation with a cuffed tube in the trachea.[198] Symptoms usually develop within six weeks of extubation but can appear up to 18 months later. Diminished effort tolerance, dyspnea, an irritative cough and the sensation of not being able to clear the throat are common. Stridor is a late feature.

Auscultation over the trachea may aid in the diagnosis and localization of a lesion, but precise information regarding its site and dimension is best obtained by air tracheogram and laminagram. Conventional contrast mediums define lesions more crisply, but they contribute little to the basic diagnosis and may precipitate acute respiratory obstruction.[199] Insufflated powdered tantalum may be a useful diagnostic tool in the future.[200] When tracheomalacia is present, intermittent narrowing of a tracheal segment may be observed with fluoroscopy and cineradiography.

In conjunction with the radiographic technics described above, bronchoscopy provides the most definitive diagnostic information. This maneuver, however, often results in increased secretions and edema, which may aggravate the existing obstruction and necessitate urgent surgical intervention. For this reason, bronchoscopy is best deferred until the time of definitive operation. Fiberoptic bronchoscopy may provide a relatively atraumatic method of tracheal inspection at an early stage.

Pathology

Trauma to the trachea from tracheostomy tubes can occur at the tip of the tube, at the level of the stoma or opposite the inflatable cuff. Among patients receiving artificial ventilation, maximal damage and deformity typically develop at the level of the inflatable cuff.[197–199] Tracheoesophageal fistula may occur or a major artery may be eroded, but this is unusual, and in the majority of cases the end result is healing with subsequent fibrosis. Although some deformity of the trachea is then common, in most cases the narrowing is minimal and of no clinical consequence.

Respiratory obstruction may be caused by polypoid granulations at the stoma. These are usually small and seldom pose any noteworthy therapeutic problems. Far more serious are the deformities of the trachea that follow more massive tissue destruction. These develop at the stoma and opposite the inflatable cuff and are often extensive and consequently far more difficult to treat.

The occurrence of lesions at the stoma is unrelated to the previous administration of artificial ventilation, and characteristically fibrosis is localized anteriorly. Causes include too large a stoma, too large a tube, excessive movements of the tube and gross local sepsis. In patients who have received artificial ventilation stenosis typically occurs 1.5 to 3 cm below the tracheostomy stoma and comprises a completely circumferential ring of fibrotic tissue, often with an associated superior segment of tracheomalacia. Histologic sections reveal varying degrees of tissue destruction. Frequently, there is grossly disturbed tracheal architecture, with completely obliterated cartilaginous rings and total absence of epithelium at the point of maximal deformity.[197,198]

Early tissue trauma at this level has been noted in all patients exposed to inflated standard cuffs for 48 hours or longer.[201] When exposure was prolonged, complete destruction and resorption of cartilage, distention of the trachea, and loss of tracheal architecture was found. In some cases, damage occurred opposite the tip of the tube, but this was relatively trivial.

Etiology

In experiments on dogs, standard inflatable cuffs produced a spectrum of tracheal lesions identical to those seen in man.[202] At the point of airtight seal, the intracuff pressure ranged from 160 to 200 mm of mercury. When specially designated large-volume, low-pressure cuffs were substituted, the intracuff pressures ranged from 20 to 40 mm of mercury, and damage was minimal. Studies in both man and dog have demonstrated that tracheal damage increases when intubation is prolonged.[199,201] Patients with tracheal stenosis and malacia seen at the Massachusetts General Hospital had received ventilatory assistance for periods varying from a few days to four months. Respiratory obstruction was more frequent, however, when ventilatory-assistance had exceeded three weeks.[1]

The influence of infection on subsequent stenosis is not clear since all tracheostomies are bacteriologically contaminated. Clinically apparent infection of the stoma was noted in some patients but did not appear to have played a part in this complication.

Impaired circulation (low cardiac output) aggravates the damage caused by pressure from the cuff. Half the patients who underwent tracheal resection for tracheal stenosis at the Massachusetts General Hospital had required vasoactive agents to support their circulation at some stage during the period in which the tracheostomy tube was in place. Among patients in cardiogenic shock and receiving circulatory support by the intra-aortic balloon technic damage at the cuff has been noted to be unusually extensive.

Prevention and treatment

The increasing number of patients receiving artificial ventilation makes prevention of tracheal stenosis an important goal. Stomal trauma can be reduced by the deployment of a swivel system of connectors at the tracheostomy.[7,198] By this means movements of the connecting tubes are buffered rather than transmitted to the tracheostomy tube. In considering lesions at a lower level, currently available information implicates pressure necrosis by the cuff as the dominant etiologic factor. Alteration of the pressure-volume characteristics appears to provide a simple and practical basis for elimination of the problem. A technic for prestretching plastic cuffs and thus producing a large-volume cuff that provides an airtight seal at reduced intracuff pressures has been described.[203] More recently clinical studies in patients who had received artificial ventilation have demonstrated a marked reduction in tracheal damage when low-pressure cuffs were employed.[204]

The treatment of symptomatic tracheal deformity depends on the site and nature of the lesion. Polypoid granulation tissue is easily amenable to bronchoscopic removal. Stenosis at the stomal site is usually secondary to scarring anteriorly, and although dilatation may help, localized resection is usually required for permanent relief of symptoms. Circumferential lesions at the cuff site are more extensive and invariably require surgical treatment. Any decision between complete surgical resection and permanent tracheostomy, however, must take into consideration the patient's general condition. With the special anesthetic and surgical technics and postoperative facilities now available, resection and anastomosis has become the treatment of choice.[199,205–207]

REFERENCES

1. Pontoppidan H, Laver MB, Geffin B: Acute respiratory failure in the surgical patient. Adv Surg 4:163–254, 1970
2. Safar P, Grenvik Å: Critical care medicine: organizing and staffing intensive care units. Chest 59:535–547, 1971
3. Weil MH, Shubin H: The new practice of critical care medicine. Chest 59:473–474, 1971
4. Bates DV, Macklem PT, Christie RV: Respiratory Function in Disease: An introduction to the integrated study of the lung. Second edition. Philadelphia, WB Saunders Company, 1971, p 442
5. Mellemgaard K: The alveolar-arterial oxygen difference: its size and components in normal man. Acta Physiol Scand 67:10–20, 1966
6. Sorbini CA, Grassi V, Solinas E, et al: Arterial oxygen tension in relation to age in healthy subjects. Respiration 25:3–13, 1968
7. Bendixen HH, Egbert LD, Hedley-Whyte J, et al: Respiratory Care. St Louis, CV Mosby Company, 1965
8. Wilson RS, Pontoppidan H: Respiratory care. Mod Med 39 (11): 100–105, 1971
9. Safar P, Grenvik Å: Multidisciplinary intensive care. Mod Med 39 (11):92–99, 1971
10. Sykes MK, McNicol MW, Campbell EJM: Respiratory Failure. Philadelphia, FA Davis Company, 1969
11. Bates DV, Macklem PT, Christie RV: Respiratory Function in Disease: An introduction to the integrated study of the lung. Second edition. Philadelphia, WB Saunders Company, 1971, pp 441–470
12. O'Donohue WJ Jr, Baker JP, Bell GM, et al: The management of acute respiratory failure in a respiratory intensive care unit. Chest 58:603–610, 1970
13. Downes JJ: Mechanical ventilation of the newborn. Anesthesiology 34:116–118, 1971
14. Wood DDW, Downes JJ, Lecks HI: The management of respiratory failure in childhood status asthmaticus: experience with 30 episodes and evolution of a technique. J Allergy 42:261–267, 1968
15. Downes JJ, Nicodemus HF, Pierce WS, et al: Acute respiratory failure in infants following cardiovascular surgery. J Thorac Cardiovasc Surg 59:21–37, 1970

References

16. Daily WJR, Sunshine P, Smith PC: Mechanical ventilation of newborn infants. V. Five years' experience. Anesthesiology 34:132–138, 1971

17. Swyer PR: Methods of artificial ventilation in the newborn (IPPV). Biol Neonate 16:3–15, 1970

18. Staub NC: The pathophysiology of pulmonary edema. Hum Pathol 1:419–432, 1970

19. Staub NC, Nagano H, Pearce ML: Pulmonary edema in dogs, especially the sequence of fluid accumulation in lungs. J Appl Physiol 22:227–240, 1967

20. Hoppin FG Jr, Green ID, Mead J: Distribution of pleural surface pressure in dogs. J Appl Physiol 27:863–873, 1969

21. Glazier JB, Hughes JMB, Maloney JE, et al: Vertical gradient of alveolar size in lungs of dogs frozen intact. J Appl Physiol 23:694–705, 1967

22. Milic-Emili J, Henderson JAM, Dolovich MB, et al: Regional distribution of inspired gas in the lung. J Appl Physiol 21:749–759, 1966

23. Sutherland PW, Katsura T, Milic-Emili J: Previous volume history of the lung and regional distribution of gas. J Appl Physiol 25:566–574, 1968

24. Hyatt RE, Okeson GC: Expiratory flow limitation, the cause of so-called "airway closure" or "closing volume." Physiologist 14:166, 1971

25. Burger EJ Jr, Macklem P: Airway closure: demonstration by breathing $100\%O_2$ at low lung volumes and by N_2 washout. J Appl Physiol 25:139–148, 1968

26. Hughes JMB, Rosenzweig DY, Kivitz PB: Site of airway closure in excised dog lungs: histologic demonstration. J Appl Physiol 29:340–344, 1970

27. Holland J, Milic-Emili J, Macklem PT, et al: Regional distribution of pulmonary ventilation and perfusion in elderly subjects. J Clin Invest 47:81–92, 1968

28. Anthonisen NR, Danson J, Robertson PC, et al: Airway closure as a function of age. Resp Physiol 8:58–65, 1969

29. Leblanc P, Ruff F, Milic-Emili J: Effects of age and body position on "airway closure" in man. J Appl Physiol 28:448–451, 1970

30. Don HF, Craig DB, Wahba WM, et al: The measurement of gas trapped in the lungs at functional residual capacity and the effects of posture. Anesthesiology 35:582–590, 1971

31. Craig DB, Wahba WM, Don HF, et al: "Closing volume" and its relationship to gas exchange in seated and supine positions. J Appl Physiol 31:717–721, 1971

32. Nunn JF, Coleman AJ, Sachithanandan T, et al: Hypoxaemia and atelectasis produced by forced expiration. Br J Anaesthesiol 37:3–12, 1965

33. Don HF, Wahba M, Cuadrado L, et al: The effects of anesthesia and 100 per cent oxygen on the functional residual capacity of the lungs. Anesthesiology 32:521–529, 1970

34. Holley HS, Milic-Emili J, Becklake MR, et al: Regional distribution of pulmonary ventilation and perfusion in obesity. J Clin Invest 46:475–481, 1967

35. Couture J, Picken J, Trop D, et al: Airway closure in normal, obese, and anesthetized supine subjects. Fed Proc 29:269, 1970

36. Hughes JMB, Rosenzweig DY: Factors affecting trapped gas volume in perfused dog lungs. J Appl Physiol 29:332–339, 1970

37. Williams JV, Tierney DF, Parker HR: Surface forces in the lung, atelectasis, and transpulmonary pressure. J Appl Physiol 21:819–827, 1966

38. Hedley-Whyte J, Berry P, Bushnell LS, et al: Effect of posture on respiratory failure, Fourth World Congress of Anaesthesiologists, London, September 9–13, 1968 (International Congress Series No. 168). Edited by TH Boulton, R Bryce-Smith, MK Sykes, et al: Amsterdam, Excerpta Medica, 1968, p 119

39. McIntyre RW, Laws AK, Ramachandran PR: Positive expiratory pressure plateau: improved gas exchange during mechanical ventilation. Can Anaesth Soc J 16:477–486, 1969

40. Kumar A, Falke KJ, Geffin B, et al: Continuous positive-pressure ventilation in acute respiratory failure: effects on hemodynamics and lung function. N Engl J Med 283:1430–1436, 1970

41. Colgan FJ, Mahoney PD: The effects of major surgery on cardiac output and shunting. Anesthesiology 31:213–221, 1969

42. Avery ME, Said S: Surface phenomena in lungs in health and disease. Medicine (Baltimore) 44:503–526, 1965

43. Clements JA: Pulmonary surfactant. Am Rev Resp Dis 101:984–990, 1970

44. Heinemann HO, Fishman AP: Nonrespiratory functions of mammalian lung. Physiol Rev 49:1–47, 1969

45. Morgan TE: Pulmonary surfactant. N Engl J Med 284:1185–1193, 1971

46. Scarpelli EM: The Surfactant System of the Lung. Philadelphia, Lea and Febiger, 1968

47. Lee C-J, Lyons JH, Konisberg S, et al: Effects of spontaneous and positive-pressure breathing of ambient air and pure oxygen at one atmosphere pressure on pulmonary surface characteristics. J Thorac Cardiovasc Surg 53:759–769, 1967

48. deLemos R, Wolfsdorf J, Nachman R, et al: Lung injury from oxygen in lambs: the role of artificial ventilation. Anesthesiology 30:609–618, 1969

49. Faridy EE, Permutt S, Riley RL: Effect of ventilation on surface forces in excised dogs' lungs. J Appl Physiol 21:1453–1462, 1966

50. Greenfield LJ, Ebert PA, Benson DW: Effect of positive pressure ventilation on surface tension properties of lung extracts. Anesthesiology 25:312–316, 1964

51. Morgan TE, Finley TN, Huber GL, et al: Alterations in pulmonary surface active lipids during exposure to increased oxygen tension. J Clin Invest 44:1737–1744, 1965

52. Pontoppidan H, Hedley-Whyte J, Bendixen HH, et al: Ventilation

References

and oxygen requirements during prolonged artificial ventilation in patients with respiratory failure. N Engl J Med 273:401–409, 1965

53. Sladen A, Laver MB, Pontoppidan H: Pulmonary complications and water retention in prolonged mechanical ventilation. N Engl J Med 279:448–453, 1968

54. Pulmonary effects of nonthoracic trauma. J Trauma 8:621–983, 1968

55. Moore FD, Lyons JH, Pierce EC, et al: Post-Traumatic Pulmonary Insufficiency: Pathophysiology of respiratory failure and principles of respiratory care after surgical operations, trauma, hemorrhage, burns and shock. Philadelphia, WB Saunders Company, 1969, pp 112–124

56. Nash G, Blennerhassett JB, Pontoppidan H: Pulmonary lesions associated with oxygen therapy and artificial ventilation. N Engl J Med 276:368–374, 1967

57. Martin AM Jr, Simmons RL, Heisterkamp CA III: Respiratory insufficiency in combat casualties. I. Pathologic changes in the lungs of patients dying of wounds. Ann Surg 170:30–38, 1969

58. Guyton AC, Lindsey AW: Effect of elevated left atrial pressure and decreased plasma protein concentration on the development of pulmonary edema. Circ Res 7:649–657, 1959

59. Levine OR, Mellins RB, Senior RM, et al: The application of Starling's law of capillary exchange to the lungs. J Clin Invest 46:934–944, 1967

60. Meyer BJ, Meyer A, Guyton AC: Interstitial fluid pressure. V. Negative pressure in the lungs. Circ Res 22:263–271, 1968

61. Permutt S, Riley RL: Hemodynamics of collapsible vessels with tone: the vascular waterfall. J Appl Physiol 18:924–932, 1963

62. West JB: Ventilation/Blood Flow and Gas Exchange. Second edition. Oxford, Blackwell Scientific Publications, 1970

63. West JB, Dollery CT, Heard BE: Increased pulmonary vascular resistance in the dependent zone of the isolated dog lung caused by perivascular edema. Circ Res 17:191–206, 1965

63a. Szidon JP, Pietra GG, Fishman AP: The alveolar-capillary membrane and pulmonary edema. Eng J Med 286:1200–1204, 1972

64. Wangensteen OD, Wittmers LE Jr, Johnson JA: Permeability of the mammalian blood-gas barrier and its components. Am J Physiol 216:719–727, 1969

65. Schneeberger-Keeley EE, Karnovsky MJ: The ultrastructural basis of alveolar-capillary membrane permeability to peroxidase used as a tracer. J Cell Biol 37:781–793, 1968

66. Pietra GG, Szidon JP, Leventhal MM, et al: Hemoglobin as a tracer in hemodynamic pulmonary edema. Science 166:1643–1646, 1969

67. Iliff LD: Extra-alveolar vessels and edema development in excised dog lungs. Circ Res 28:524–532, 1971

68. Cottrell TS, Levine OR, Senior RM, et al: Electron microscopic alterations at the alveolar level in pulmonary edema. Circ Res 21:783–797, 1967

69. Michalski AH, Lowenstein E, Austen WG, et al: Patterns of oxygenation and cardiovascular adjustment to acute, transient normovolemic anemia. Ann Surg 168:946–956, 1968
70. Said SI, Longacher JW Jr, Davis RK, et al: Pulmonary gas exchange during induction of pulmonary edema in anesthetized dogs. J Appl Physiol 19:403–407, 1964
71. Ruff F, Hughes JMB, Stanley N, et al: Regional lung function in patients with hepatic cirrhosis. J Clin Invest 50:2403–2413, 1971
72. Levine OR, Mellins RB, Fishman AP: Quantitative assessment of pulmonary edema. Circ Res 17:414–426, 1965
73. Chinard FP, Enns T: Transcapillary pulmonary exchange of water in the dog. Am J Physiol 178:197–202, 1954
74. Lowenstein E, Travis K, Malt RA, et al: Substitution of iodoantipyrine-I[131] (IAP) for H[3]O in the pulmonary extra vascular water (PEVW) measurement. Fed Proc 28:281, 1969
75. McCredie M: Measurement of pulmonary edema in valvular heart disease. Circulation 36:381–386, 1967
76. Turino GM, Edelman NH, Senior RM, et al: Extravascular lung water in cor pulmonale. Bull Physio-Pathol Resp 4:47–64, 1968
77. Gump FE, Mashima Y, Kinney JM: Water balance and extravascular lung water measurements in surgical patients. Am J Surg 119:515–518, 1970
78. Goresky CA, Cronin RFP, Wangel BE: Indicator dilution measurements of extravascular water in the lungs. J Clin Invest 48:487–501, 1969
79. Kilburn KH, Dowell AR: Renal function in respiratory failure: effects of hypoxia, hyperoxia, and hypercapnia. Arch Intern Med 127:754–762, 1971
80. Posner JB, Ertel NH, Kossmann RJ, et al: Hyponatremia in acute polyneuropathy: four cases with the syndrome of inappropriate secretion of antidiuretic hormone. Arch Neurol 17:530–541, 1967
81. Bartter FC, Schwartz WB: The syndrome of inappropriate secretion of antidiuretic hormone. Am J Med 42:790–806, 1967
81a. Khambatta HJ, Baratz RA: IPPB, plasma ADH, and urine flow in conscious man. J Appl Physiol 33:362–364, 1972
82. Philbin DM, Baratz RA, Patterson RW: The effect of carbon dioxide on plasma antidiuretic hormone levels during intermittent positive-pressure breathing. Anesthesiology 33:345–349, 1970
83. Skillman JJ, Parikh BM, Tanenbaum BJ: Pulmonary arteriovenous admixture: improvement with albumin and diuresis. Am J Surg 119:440–447, 1970
84. Swan HJC, Ganz W, Forrester J, et al: Catheterization of the heart in man with use of a flow-directed balloon-tipped catheter. N Engl J Med 283:447–451, 1970
85. Nunn JF: Applied Respiratory Physiology With Special Reference to Anaesthesia. New York, Appleton-Century-Crofts, 1969
86. West JB:[62] p 100
87. *Idem:*[62] p 108
88. Hedley-Whyte J, Pontoppidan H, Morris MJ: The response of

patients with respiratory failure and cardiopulmonary disease to different levels of constant volume ventilation. J Clin Invest 45: 1543–1554, 1966

89. West JB: Causes of carbon dioxide retention in lung disease. N Engl J Med 284:1232–1236, 1971

90. Prys-Roberts C, Kelman GR, Greenbaum R: The influence of circulatory factors on arterial oxygenation during anaesthesia in man. Anaesthesia 22:257–275, 1967

91. Philbin DM, Sullivan SF, Bowman FO Jr, et al: Postoperative hypoxemia: contribution of the cardiac output. Anesthesiology 32:136–142, 1970

92. Michenfelder JD, Fowler WS, Theye RA: CO_2 levels and pulmonary shunting in anesthetized man. J Appl Physiol 21:1471–1476, 1966

93. Sanders CA, Harthorne JW, Heitman H, et al: Effect of vasopressor administration on blood gas exchange in mitral disease. Clin Res 13:351, 1965

94. Penman RWB, Howard P, Stentiford NH: Factors influencing pulmonary gas exchange in patients with acute edematous cor pulmonale due to chronic lung disease. Am J Med 44:8–15, 1968

95. Finch CA, Lenfant C: Oxygen transport in man. N Engl J Med 286:407–415, 1972

96. McConn R, Del Guercio LRM: Respiratory function of blood in the acutely ill patient and the effect of steroids. Ann Surg 174:436–450, 1971

97. Broennle AM, Laver MB, Huggins C, et al: Oxygen transport and massive transfusion: the unsteady state. Surg Forum 21:52–53, 1970

98. Clark JM, Lambertsen CJ: Pulmonary oxygen toxicity: a review. Pharmacol Rev 23:37–133, 1971

99. Caldwell PRB, Lee WL Jr, Schildkraut HS, et al: Changes in lung volume, diffusing capacity, and blood gases in men breathing oxygen. J Appl Physiol 21:1477–1483, 1966

100. Fisher AB, Hyde RW, Puy RJM, et al: Effect of oxygen at 2 atmospheres on the pulmonary mechanics of normal man. J Appl Physiol 24:529–536, 1968

101. Puy RJM, Hyde RW, Fisher AB, et al: Alterations in the pulmonary capillary bed during early O_2 toxicity in man. J Appl Physiol 24:537–543, 1968

102. Singer MM, Wright F, Stanley LK, et al: Oxygen toxicity in man: a prospective study in patients after open-heart surgery. N Engl J Med 283:1473–1478, 1970

103. Barber RE, Lee J, Hamilton WK: Oxygen toxicity in man: a prospective study in patients with irreversible brain damage. N Engl J Med 283:1478–1484, 1970

104. Kaplan HP, Robinson FR, Kapanci Y, et al: Pathogenesis and reversibility of the pulmonary lesions of oxygen toxicity in monkeys. I. Clinical and light microscopic studies. Lab Invest 20:94–100, 1969

105. Kapanci Y, Weibel ER, Kaplan HP, et al: Pathogenesis and re-

versibility of the pulmonary lesions of oxygen toxicity in monkeys. II. Ultrastructural and morphometric studies. Lab Invest 20:101–118, 1969

106. Nash G, Bowen JA, Langlinais PC: "Respirator lung": a misnomer. Arch Pathol 91:234–240, 1971

107. Winter PM, Gupta RK, Michalski AH, et al: Modification of hyperbaric oxygen toxicity by experimental venous admixture. J Appl Physiol 23:954–963, 1967

108. Miller WW, Waldhausen JA, Rashkind WJ: Comparison of oxygen poisoning of the lung in cyanotic and acyanotic dogs. N Engl J Med 282:943–947, 1970

109. Northway WH Jr, Rosan RC, Porter DY: Pulmonary disease following respirator therapy of hyaline-membrane disease: bronchopulmonary dysplasia. N Engl J Med 276:357–368, 1967

110. Laurenzi GA, Yin S, Guarneri JJ: Adverse effect of oxygen on tracheal mucus flow. N Engl J Med 279:333–339, 1968

111. Hyde RW, Rawson AJ: Unintentional iatrogenic oxygen pneumonitis—response to therapy. Ann Intern Med 71:517–531, 1969

112. Hedley-Whyte J, Winter PM: Oxygen therapy. Clin Pharmacol Ther 8:696–737, 1967

113. Wright RA, Weiss HS, Hiatt EP, et al: Risk of mortality in interrupted exposure to 100% O_2: role of air vs. lowered Po_2. Am J Physiol 210:1015–1020, 1966

114. Fairley HB, Britt BA: The adequacy of the air-mix control in ventilators operated from an oxygen source. Can Med Assoc J 90:1394–1396, 1964

115. Pontoppidan H, Berry PR: Regulation of the inspired oxygen concentration during artificial ventilation. JAMA 201:11–14, 1967

116. Norlander OP: The use of respirators in anaesthesia and surgery. Acta Anaesthesiol Scand (Suppl) 30:1–74, 1968

117. Comroe JH Jr, Forster RE II, DuBois AB, et al: The Lung: Clinical physiology and pulmonary function tests. Second edition. Chicago, Year Book Medical Publishers, 1962, p 194

118. Grenvik Å: Respiratory, circulatory and metabolic effects of respirator treatment: a clinical study in postoperative thoracic surgical patients. Acta Anaesthesiol Scand (Suppl) 19:1–122, 1966

119. Garzon AA, Seltzer B, Karlson KE: Physiopathology of crushed chest injuries. Ann Surg 168:128–136, 1968

120. Wilson RS, Sullivan SF, Malm JR, et al: The postoperative cost of breathing. Clin Res 18:493, 1970

121. Berry PR, Pontoppidan H: Oxygen consumption and blood gas exchange during controlled and spontaneous ventilation in patients with respiratory failure. Anesthesiology 29:177–178, 1968

122. Bay J, Nunn JF, Prys-Roberts C: Factors influencing arterial Po_2 during recovery from anaesthesia. Br J Anaesth 40:398–407, 1968

123. Riley RL: The work of breathing and its relation to respiratory acidosis. Ann Intern Med 41:172–176, 1954

124. Bendixen HH, Laver MB: Hypoxia in anesthesia: a review. Clin Pharmacol Ther 6:510–539, 1965

103

References

125. Darling RC: Ruptured arteriosclerotic abdominal aortic aneurysms: a pathologic and clinical study. Amer J Surg 119:397–401, 1970.

126. Laver MB: Prevention of postoperative respiratory complications, Complications of Anesthesia. Edited by LJ Saidman, F Moya. Springfield, Illinois, Charles C Thomas, 1970, pp 31–39

127. Williams MH Jr, Shim CS: Ventilatory failure: etiology and clinical forms. Am J Med 48:477–483, 1970

128. Klein RL, Safar P, Grenvik Å: Respiratory care in blunt chest injury—retrospective review of 43 cases. Abstracts of Scientific Papers, Annual Meeting of American Society of Anesthesiologists, New York, October 17–21, 1970, pp 145–146

129. Plum F, Brown HW: The effect on respiration of central nervous system disease. Ann NY Acad Sci 109:915–931, 1963

130. Gordon E: The acid-base balance and oxygen tension of the cerebrospinal fluid, and their implications for the treatment of patients with brain lesions. Acta Anaesthesiol Scand (Suppl) 39:1–36, 1971

131. Avery WG, Samet P, Sackner MA: The acidosis of pulmonary edema. Am J Med 48:320–324, 1970

132. Moore FD, Lyons JH, Pierce EC, et al: Post-Traumatic Pulmonary Insufficiency: Pathophysiology of respiratory failure and principles of respiratory care after surgical operations, trauma, hemorrhage, burns and shock. Philadelphia, WB Saunders Company, 1969, p 125

133. Burke JF, Pontoppidan H, Welch CE: High output respiratory failure: an important cause of death ascribed to peritonitis or ileus. Ann Surg 158:581–595, 1963

134. Freedman S, Campbell EJM: The ability of normal subjects to tolerate added inspiratory loads. Resp Physiol 10:213–235, 1970

135. Yakaitis RW, Cooke JE, Redding JS: Re-evaluation of relationships of hyperkalemia and Pco_2 to cardiac arrhythmias during mechanical ventilation. Anesth Analg (Cleve) 50:368–373, 1971

136. Rotheram EB Jr, Safar P, Robin ED: CNS disorder during mechanical ventilation in chronic pulmonary disease JAMA 189:993–996, 1964

137. Kilburn KH: Shock, seizures, and coma with alkalosis during mechanical ventilation. Ann Intern Med 65:977–984, 1966

138. Rie MW: Physical therapy in the nursing care of respiratory disease patients. Nurs Clin North Am 3:463–478, 1968

139. Noble MIM, Trenchard D, Guz A: The value of diuretics in respiratory failure. Lancet 2:257–260, 1966

139a. Baum GL, Schwartz A, Llamas R, Castillo C: Left ventricular function in chronic obstructive lung disease. N Engl J Med 285:361–365, 1971

140. Eldridge F, Gherman C: Studies of oxygen administration in respiratory failure. Ann Intern Med 68:569–578, 1968

141. Petty TL: Intensive and Rehabilitative Respiratory Care. Philadelphia, Lea and Febiger, 1971, pp 102–121

142. Asmundsson T, Kilburn KH: Survival of acute respiratory failure: a study of 239 episodes. Ann Intern Med 70:471–485, 1969
143. Sykes MK, McNicol MW, Campbell EJM:[10] pp 252–256
144. McFadden ER Jr, Lyons HA: Arterial-blood gas tension in asthma. N Engl J Med 278:1027–1032, 1968
145. Gold MI, Helrich M: Pulmonary mechanics during general anesthesia. V. Status asthmaticus. Anesthesiology 32:422–428, 1970
146. Ambiavagar M, Jones ES: Resuscitation of the moribund asthmatic: use of intermittent positive pressure ventilation, bronchial lavage and intravenous infusions. Anaesthesia 22:375–391, 1967
147. Finley TN, Swenson EW, Curran WS, et al: Bronchopulmonary lavage in normal subjects and patients with obstructive lung disease. Ann Intern Med 66:651–658, 1967
148. Rogers RM, Szidon JP, Shelburne J, et al: Hemodynamic response of the pulmonary circulation to bronchopulmonary lavage in man. N Engl J Med 286:1230–1233, 1972
149. Lefemine AA, Browning, JR, Stewart SK: Bronchoscopy and bronchial lavage for obstructive ventilatory insufficiency. Ann Thorac Surg 4:308–318, 1967
150. Cournand A, Motley HL, Werko L, et al: Physiological studies of the effects of intermittent positive pressure breathing on cardiac output in man. Am J Physiol 152:162–174, 1948
151. Guyton AC: Circulatory Physiology: Cardiac output and its regulation. Philadelphia, WB Saunders Company, 1963, pp 380–383
152. Morgan BC, Crawford EW, Guntheroth WG: The hemodynamic effects of changes in blood volume during intermittent positive-pressure ventilation. Anesthesiology 30:297–305, 1969
153. Prys-Roberts C, Kelman GR, Greenbaum R, et al: Circulatory influences of artificial ventilation during nitrous oxide anesthesia in man. II. Results: the relative influence of mean intrathoracic pressure and arterial carbon dioxide tension. Br J Anaesth 39:533–548, 1967
154. Uzawa T, Ashbaugh DG: Continuous positive-pressure breathing in acute hemorrhagic pulmonary edema. J Appl Physiol 26:427–432, 1969
155. Falke KJ, Pontoppidan H, Kumar A, et al: Ventilation with end-expiratory pressure in acute lung disease. J Clin Invest 51:2315–2323, 1972
156. Cullen DJ, Eger EI II, Gregory GA: The cardiovascular effects of carbon dioxide in man, conscious and during cyclopropane anesthesia. Anesthesiology 31:407–413, 1969
157. Mead J, Whittenberger JL: Lung inflation and hemodynamics, Handbook of Physiology: A critical, comprehensive presentation of physiological knowledge and concepts. Section 3, Respiration. Vol. 1. Section editors WO Fenn, H Rahn. Washington, DC, American Physiological Society, 1964, pp 477–486
158. West JB: Effects of interstitial pressure. The Pulmonary Circulation and Interstitial Space. Edited by AP Fishman, HH Hecht. Chicago, University of Chicago Press, 1969, pp 43–63

References

159. The Pulmonary Circulation and Interstitial Space. Edited by AP Fishman, HH Hecht. Chicago, University of Chicago Press, 1969.
160. Mead J, Collier C: Relation of volume history of lungs to respiratory mechanics in anesthetized dogs. J Appl Physiol 14:669–678, 1959
161. Bendixen HH, Hedley-Whyte J, Laver MB: Impaired oxygenation in surgical patients during general anesthesia with controlled ventilation: a concept of atelectasis. N Engl J Med 269:991–996, 1963
162. Laver MB, Morgan J Bendixen HH, et al: Lung volume, compliance, and arterial oxygen tensions during controlled ventilation. J Appl Physiol 19:725–733, 1964
163. Bergman NA: Concerning sweet dreams, health, and quiet breathing. Anesthesiology 32:297–298, 1970
164. Hedley-Whyte J, Pontoppidan H, Laver MB, et al: Arterial oxygenation during hypothermia. Anesthesiology 26:595–602, 1965
165. Suwa K, Geffin B, Pontoppidan H, et al: A nomogram for dead-space requirement during prolonged artificial ventilation. Anesthesiology 29:1206–1210, 1968
166. Knelson JH, Howatt WF, DeMuth GR: Effect of respiratory pattern on alveolar gas exchange. J Appl Physiol 29:328–331, 1970
167. Lyager S: Ventilation/perfusion ratio during intermittent positive-pressure ventilation: importance of no-flow interval during the insufflation. Acta Anaesthesiol Scand 14:211–232, 1970
168. Barach AL: Principles and Practices of Inhalation Therapy. Philadelphia, JB Lippincott Company, 1944, pp 52-57
169. Gregory GA, Kitterman JA, Phibbs RH, et al: Treatment of the idiopathic respiratory-distress syndrome with continuous positive airway pressure. N Engl J Med 284:1333–1340, 1971
170. Frumin MJ, Bergman NA, Holaday DA, et al: Alveolar-arterial O_2 differences during artificial respiration in man. J Appl Physiol 14:694–700, 1959
171. Ashbaugh DG, Petty TL, Bigelow DB, et al: Continuous positive-pressure breathing (CPPB) in adult respiratory distress syndrome. J Thorac Cardiovasc Surg 57:31–41, 1969
172. Hughes JMB, Glazier JB, Maloney JE, et al: Effect of lung volume on the distribution of pulmonary blood flow in man. Resp Physiol 4:58–72, 1968
173. Laver MB, Hallowell P, Goldblatt A: Pulmonary dysfunction secondary to heart disease: aspects relevant to anesthesia and surgery. Anesthesiology 33:161–192, 1970
174. Radford EP Jr: Ventilation standards for use in artificial respiration. J Appl Physiol 7:451–460, 1955
175. Askrog V: Changes in (a-A)CO_2 difference and pulmonary artery pressure in anesthetized man. J Appl Physiol 21:1299–1305, 1966
176. Sykes, MK, Adams AP, Finlay WEI, et al: The effects of variations in end-expiratory inflation pressure on cardiorespiratory function in normo-, hypo- and hypervolaemic dogs. Br J Anaesth 42:669–677, 1970
177. Parsons EF, Travis K, Shore N, et al: Effect of positive pressure

breathing on distribution of pulmonary blood flow and ventilation. Am Rev Resp Dis 103:356–361, 1971

178. Prolonged endotracheal intubation. Br Med J 1:321–322, 1967
179. Hatcher CR Jr: Prolonged endotracheal intubation. Ann Thorac Surg 5:478–480, 1968
180. Pilcher J: Prolonged orotracheal intubation without tracheostomy for respiratory failure. Br J Dis Chest 61:95–100, 1967
181. Rees GJ, Owen-Thomas JB: A technique of pulmonary ventilation with a nasotracheal tube. Br J Anaesth 38:901–906, 1966
182. Allen TH, Steven IM: Prolonged endotracheal intubation in infants and children. Br J Anaesth 37:566–573, 1965
183. Bergström J, Moberg A, Orell SR: On the pathogenesis of laryngeal injuries following prolonged intubation. Acta Otolaryngol (Stockh) 55:342–346, 1962
184. Harrison GA, Tonkin JP: Prolonged (therapeutic) endotracheal intubation. Br J Anaesth 40:241–249, 1968
185. Bergström J: Laryngologic aspects of the treatment of acute barbiturate poisoning. Acta Otolaryngol [Suppl] (Stockh) 173:1–59, 1962
186. Brandstater B: Prolonged intubation: an alternative to tracheostomy in infants, First European Congress of Anaesthesiology: Proceedings. Vienna, World Federation of Societies of Anaesthesiologists, 1962, p 106
187. Harrison GA, Tonkin JP: Laryngeal complications of prolonged endotracheal intubation. Med J Aust 2:709–710, 1965
188. Tonkin JP, Harrison GA: The effect on the larynx of prolonged endotracheal intubation. Med J Aust 2:581–587, 1966
189. Dwyer CS, Kronenberg S, Saklad M: The endotracheal tube: a consideration of its traumatic effects with a suggestion for the modification thereof. Anesthesiology 10:714–728, 1949
190. Way WL, Sooy FA: Histologic changes produced by endotracheal intubation. Ann Otol Rhinol Laryngol 74:799–812, 1965
191. Striker TW, Stool S, Downes JJ: Prolonged nasotracheal intubation in infants and children. Arch Otolaryngol 85:210–213, 1967
192. Guess WL, Stetson JB: Tissue reactions to organotin-stabilized polyvinyl chloride (PVC) catheters. JAMA 204:580–584, 1968
193. Little K, Parkhouse J: Tissue reactions to polymers. Lancet 2:857–861, 1962
194. Cunliffe, AC, Wesley F: Hazards from plastics sterilized by ethylene oxide. Br Med J 2:575–576, 1967
195. Matsumoto T, Hardaway RM III, Pani KC, et al: Safe standard of aeration for ethylene oxide sterilized supplies. Arch Surg 96:464–470, 1968
196. Stetson JB, Guess WL: Cause of damage to tissues by polymers and elastomers used in the fabrication of tracheal devices. Anesthesiology 33:635–652, 1970
197. Pearson FG, Goldberg M, da Silva AJ. Tracheal stenosis complicating tracheostomy with cuffed tubes: clinical experience and observations from a prospective study. Arch Surg 97:380–394, 1968

References

198. Geffin B, Grillo HC, Cooper JD, et al: Stenosis following tracheostomy for respiratory care. JAMA 216:1984–1988, 1971
199. Grillo HC: The management of tracheal stenosis following assisted respiration. J Thorac Cardiovasc Surg 57:52–71, 1969
200. Nadel JA, Wolfe WG, Graf PD: Powdered tantalum as a medium for bronchography in canine and human lungs. Invest Radiol 3:229–238, 1968
201. Cooper JD, Grillo HC: The evolution of tracheal injury due to ventilatory assistance through cuffed tubes: a pathologic study. Ann Surg 169:334–348, 1969
202. *Idem:* Experimental production and prevention of injury due to cuffed tracheal tubes. Surg Gynecol Obstet 129:1235–1241, 1969
203. Geffin B, Pontoppidan H: Reduction of tracheal damage by the prestretching of inflatable cuffs. Anesthesiology 31:462–463, 1969
204. Grillo HC, Cooper JD, Geffin B, et al: A low-pressure cuff for tracheostomy tubes to minimize tracheal injury: a comparative clinical trial. J Thorac Cardiovasc Surg 62:898–907, 1971
205. Geffin B, Bland J, Grillo HC: Anesthetic management of tracheal resection and reconstruction. Anesth Analg (Cleve) 48:884–894, 1969
206. Grillo HC: Circumferential resection and reconstruction of the mediastinal and cervical trachea. Ann Surg 162:374–388, 1965
207. Grillo HC, Bendixen HH, Gephart T: Resection of the carina and lower trachea. Ann Surg 158:889–893, 1963

INDEX

Adhesions, endotracheal intubation and, 91

Airway(s)
closure, 6, 12, 13, 15–16
age and, 10, 11
alveolar closure vs., 13–15
atelectasis and, 12
breathing at low lung volume and, 13
closing volume and, 9, 11
gas distribution and, 11–12
at inspiration, 9
oxygen breathing and, 53
positive end-expiratory pressure and, 83
obstruction, oxygen cost of breathing and, 59–60
open, at inspiration, 9
pressure
cardiac output and, 72–74
positive end-expiratory pressure and, 72

Albumin, diuresis plus, in pulmonary edema, 32

Alloxan, pulmonary edema and, 21

Alveolar-arterial oxygen gradient, 62
in acute pulmonary disease, 63
artificial ventilation duration and, 77–78
cardiac output and, 42–43
controlled ventilation and, 77–78
factors determining, 39–42
hypoxemia and, 53–54
as measurement of efficiency of oxygen exchange, 37, 38, 39, 40, 41
in obstructive pulmonary disease, 41–42
tidal volume and, 77–78

Alveolar carbon dioxide tension, ventilation-perfusion ratio and, 40

Alveolar oxygen tension. See also Alveolar-arterial oxygen gradient
closing volume and, 12
determination, 39
right-to-left shunt and, 38

Alveoli
closure, 6, 15, 16. See also Closing volume
airway closure vs., 13–15
collapse
in obstructive vs. nonobstructive pulmonary disease, 65
positive end-expiratory pressure and, 83
gas distribution to, in normal breathing, 8, 9
in inspiration, 9
oxygen breathing and, 51, 53
permeability of, 21, 25
pressure, 7, 9
in pulmonary edema, 21, 26
size, factors affecting, 7, 9
surfactant and, 16, 18

Anesthesia
alveolar-arterial oxygen gradient and right-to-left shunt and, 43
use, in status asthmaticus, 66–67

109

Index

Arterial carbon dioxide tension, 2
in bronchial asthma, 66
cardiac output and, 74–75
controlled hyperventilation and,
62
functional residual capacity and,
15
intermittent positive-pressure
ventilation and, 83
mechanical ventilation and, 65,
74–75
minute ventilation and, 86
pulmonary water and, 65
Arterial oxygen tension. *See also*
Alveolar-arterial oxygen
gradient; Oxygenation
age and, 2, 10, 12
blood flow and, 45
closing volume and, 12
functional residual capacity and,
15
hemoglobin dissociation curve
and, 65
inspiratory flow pattern and, 78
inspired oxygen and, 37, 38, 39–
42, 55, 63, 64
oxygen breathing and, 49–51
physiologic information and, 35,
37
positive end-expiratory pressure
and, 44, 72, 81, 82–83, 84–85
range in acute respiratory failure, 2
right-to-left shunt and, 37, 38,
55, 63, 64
transpulmonary pressure and
lung volume and, 15
"true physiologic" shunt, 40, 41
Antidiuretic hormone (ADH) secretion, 30–31
Artificial airways. *See* Endotracheal intubation; Tracheostomy
Artificial ventilation. *See* Mechanical ventilation
Asthma, 66–67
Atelectasis
airway closure and, 12
compliance and, 12

oxygen breathing and absorption, 53
pathogenesis, 62
"physiologic," 26
vital capacity and, 65
Auscultation of tracheal lesions,
93

Blood flow. *See* Circulation
Blood volume
cardiac output and, 71, 74
mechanical ventilation and, 70
replacement requirements, 33
Breathing. *See also* Expiration;
Inspiration; Mechanical
ventilation; Oxygen breathing; Positive end-expiratory
pressure (PEEP)
continuous positive-pressure
plus spontaneous, 79
gas distribution in normal, 8, 9
intermittent positive-pressure.
See Intermittent positive-
pressure ventilation (IPPV)
at low lung volume, 12, 13
in obstructive pulmonary disease, 59–60
oxygen consumption in, 58–59
respiratory muscles in, 46–48
tolerance to ventilatory work
load, 59
work of, 58–60, 63
Bronchial asthma, 66–67
Bronchial lavage, 66–67
Bronchodilators for obstructive
pulmonary disease, 60
Bronchoscopy in tracheal lesion
diagnosis, 93

Capillaries. *See* Transcapillary exchange
Carbon dioxide
removal, in mechanical ventilation, 69, 86
tension. *See* Alveolar carbon dioxide tension, ventilation-
perfusion ratio and; Ar-
terial carbon dioxide tension